D1071347

FOR BETTER OR FOR WORSE

A COUPLE'S GUIDE TO DEALING WITH CHRONIC ILLNESS

BEVERLY KIEVMAN
with Susie Blackmun

CB
CONTEMPORARY
BOOKS
CHICAGO · NEW YORK

Library of Congress Cataloging-in-Publication Data

Kievman, Beverly, 1937–
    For better or for worse : a couple's guide to dealing with
chronic illness / Beverly Kievman with Susie Blackmun.
        p.   cm.
    Bibliography: p.
    ISBN 0-8092-4600-7 : $17.95
    1. Chronically ill—Family relationships.   2. Chronically ill—
Home care—Psychological aspects.   I. Blackmun, Susie.
II. Title.
RC108.K49   1989
616—dc19   89-30688
                                                                    CIP

Published by Contemporary Books, Inc.
180 North Michigan Avenue, Chicago, Illinois 60601
Manufactured in the United States of America
Library of Congress Catalog Card Number: 89-30688
International Standard Book Number: 0-8092-4600-7

Published simultaneously in Canada by Beaverbooks, Ltd.
195 Allstate Parkway, Valleywood Business Park
Markham, Ontario L3R 4T8 Canada

Contents

This book is lovingly dedicated to the memory of Michael Kievman, whose strong will and determination were an inspiration, and to the cherished memory of my mom, Bess Segal Stein.

Acknowledgments

I wish to express my deep gratitude to the following people:

Susie Blackmun, my talented and caring collaborator, who forced me to focus on the messages that *you* needed to know rather than the hurt, sadness, anger, and negative feelings that mattered only to me. The sensitivity that she exhibited with me, as well as during the numerous interviews, gave me encouragement through many dark days when I had no more words inside me.

Diane C. Thomas, who played a key role in bringing this book to fruition by producing a workable outline, setting the tone for the book, finding resources, drafting Chapters 1, 5, 6, and 11, and keeping us organized; Faye Goolrick for drafting Chapter 9; and Mark Mayer for supplying research and draft material.

J. R. Beahrs, M.D.; Donna Barwick, J.D.; Sally Blackmun, J.D.; Peter W. Carryer, M.D.; John C. Coniaris, M.D.; Nancy B. Coniaris, Psy.D.; Donna Hamer; Connie D. Hill; Sally T. Lehr, R.N., M.N.; James L. Mammoser; Kathy Newman, R.N., B.S.N.; Mary Ann Outwater; Jeanne Shaw, Ph.D.; Kitty Stein, Psy.D.; William C. Talmadge, Ph.D.; Linda E. Van Tuyl, R.N., M.S.; and Jack H. Watson, Jr., Esq., for supplying us with professional information and advice.

The children, especially Michele, Mark, Corin, and Steven, who helped me remember.

My loving and supportive family and friends, who kept encouraging and bugging me the many times I stalled out, especially my dad, Jack Stein; Robin Stein, Kathy Ray, Mark Needle, Jack Watson, Elizabeth Ryon Sampsell, and Eddie Robinson; Sylvia, Sid, Mel, Jannie, Sharon, Sam, Jan, Greg, Adella, and Sis; two special doctors, John Leonardy and David Rosenthal; Carole Hyatt, who planted the seed in my head; Julia Coopersmith; and our editor, Bernie Shir-Cliff.

The many caregivers and patients who gave freely of their hearts, both in pain and in victory, especially Marie, Pat, Arlene, and Ann.

Everyone involved in Mike's Night, especially Bill Schwartz, John Furman, Pat Gmiter, Tim Hughes, Jerry Freeman, and all 250 friends who attended.

A portion of the proceeds of this book will be donated to the Stein/Kievman Foundation.

Prologue

O ne day I was a happy-go-lucky, loved, and highly motivated individual. I was married to a terrific, respected person, we had six children (collectively), and my own career was ready to blossom to a new level of success. Two years later, slowly and insidiously, everything had changed. My world was hanging by a narrow thread through circumstances totally out of my control.

Let me give you an analogy to describe how I felt. When a hockey player commits a foul, he is penalized for an exact length of time—two minutes, for example—and sent into the penalty box. From there he can watch the action going on, but he is out of the game until his penalty time is up. Ironically, in the game of life we may not ever commit a foul, yet we find ourselves in the penalty box. Dr. Bill Self says:

> Life has a way of putting us in the penalty box. It is a human dilemma for each of us; it could be a business disappointment, a marriage failure, growing old, illness, or one of a hundred things. What do you do when you are out of the game?

You have picked up this book because you are reaching out for help for yourself, a loved one, or a friend. That is probably the single most important thing you can do at this moment. If you or someone you love is in the penalty box right now, it is likely going to be a long time before you are back in the game. The real question is what can you do to regain control of your life during this time?

I have shared my private thoughts and feelings openly in hopes that my experiences of the past five years will make your life more meaningful. Of even more importance, Susie Blackmun and I have talked with dozens of caregivers and patients who shared their own intimate feelings and lives with us; some of them had never expressed these thoughts to another person.

In our research we found several distinct categories of caregivers, ranging from those who tried to deny that their spouse was ill to those who were definitely in control and felt quite on top of their situation. The majority, however, were in the middle—going through a very tough time, in emotional pain themselves, feeling very much alone, and eager for positive ideas or help. Gathering the information in this book has required the expenditure of enormous amounts of time and energy by a dynamic team of people. The synergy generated by the combination of our unique perspectives has enhanced the depth of the stories and their presentation. I could not have done it alone.

But perhaps that is the essence of dealing with chronic illness. One person cannot do it alone. While waiting until my time in the penalty box was over, the inspiration came to me to use the time to help and serve other people in need. A dear friend helped me to see how this book should be written. All of us offer the fruits of our labor to you.

PART I
FEELINGS,
EMOTIONS,
RELATIONSHIPS

1
When Your Life Partner Becomes Chronically Ill

M ichael was gorgeous. That was what I thought the first time I saw him in the Jezebel, a piano bar that is a favorite gathering place for Atlanta's business professionals. In a room filled with forceful, attractive people, Michael was a standout.

It was close to the holidays, and the atmosphere was very Christmassy. Although both of us had come with someone else, before long we were introduced. For more than an hour we talked as though we were the only people in the room. I have associated a song that was popular then, "The First Time Ever I Saw Your Face (I Felt the Earth Move in My Hand)," with that evening ever since.

Michael was the vice-president in charge of programming for Cox Broadcasting and a major figure in the broadcasting industry. At one point he was chairman of the board that enforced the standards code of the National Association of Broadcasters. He always stood behind what he believed in and was never afraid to take a risk for it.

I was the owner of a modeling and talent agency and one of the city's most visible female entrepreneurs. We made a dynamic couple, and for a while our whirlwind lives made me feel like the heroine in a fairy tale. We bought a house on Grand Cayman Island, and we spent as much time there as we could. Our vacations were always filled with friends and good fellowship. Michael fished, snorkeled, and played cards, and the two of us walked on the beach for miles.

One day he couldn't walk as far because his legs hurt. Diabetes, which had severely afflicted both his parents, was now bearing down hard on their son. Michael had always been a fighter, but this was one battle he would not be able to win. The disease caught up with him, took both his legs, and made this powerful man dependent. For the last four years of his life, I was his caregiver.

How This Book Began

In January 1987 Michael lay unconscious in a hospital. He had survived against great odds a life-or-death operation to remove his second leg. His doctors had agreed that there was nothing more they could do for him. I said, "All right, then, I want to take him home."

Now I stood on the deck of our house, counting the steps I had just climbed and staring with a growing sense of hopelessness at a door that was too narrow for a wheelchair to pass through. Then I thought about the bathroom and the other rooms that would be inaccessible to anyone who was wheelchair bound, and it hit me that what I had set out to do might not even be possible.

In business I had always had a mentor, someone I could turn to for advice and encouragement. There was no one I knew who could serve as my mentor now. I would have to go this one alone.

"Forever" stretched out in front of me like a long, gray road that continued beyond the distant horizon. I looked down that road and despaired of what would happen to my career, feeling horribly ashamed of myself for even thinking about such a thing at such a time. But I couldn't help wondering what would happen to my life and whether I would ever have any time alone to call my own again. I despaired over what the rest of Michael's life might be like and wondered how I was going to get through it. But most of all I bitterly missed the well Michael who had been my husband, lover, and best friend. I went inside the house, closed the door, sank down on the sofa, and screamed.

Then I cried.

When I had finished crying, I took out the notebook I always carried with me. I had gotten the panic and tears out of my system, at least for now. It was time to get practical.

I wrote down everything I could think of that needed to be changed inside the house so that Michael could function there. I noted what had to be done immediately and what could be done a few days or weeks later. All the time I kept thinking, as I had so many times before, what a help and comfort it would be to know someone who had already gone through what I was going through at this moment. How wonderful it would be to have someone provide me with a checklist of all I needed to do and explain my available options. Even more importantly, I wanted someone I could share my feelings with, especially the ones I acknowledged only in my secret notebook because they sounded so horrible and selfish that I was afraid no one would understand.

Not knowing where to turn, I searched bookstores for anything that could help explain what we were going through. I found books on death and dying and on caring for a patient at home, but nowhere did I find any help on coping with a loved one who goes through a painful transition from the person you married, for better or for worse, to someone totally different—for the rest of your life together.

Out of that frustration came the idea for this book. It would be a guide for people whose life partners are handicapped or the victims of stroke, who suffer from Alzheimer's disease, lupus, multiple sclerosis, lung disease, cancer, or any other chronically debilitating condition. It would deal with the emotional aspects of the situation and with the practical side as well.

We conducted dozens of interviews, both with caregivers and with their chronically ill mates. I wanted to find out how they adjusted to their new situations, how they lived from day to day, and what attitudes or personality traits helped them get by. In a sense, I have tried to create for others the mentor whom I so often wished for yet did not have.

I have always been an optimist. My glass is never half empty; it is always half full. During much of Michael's illness I was starting a new business that involved several major outside investors. At one point two close friends and business colleagues, concerned about whether I was holding up under the strain of functioning both as Michael's caregiver and as the force behind the fledgling business, recommended that I pay a visit to a friend of theirs, a psychiatrist practicing in New York. I did. I spent two hours with her, and she was a wonderful person to talk to. At the end of the session she said the most reassuring words I could have wanted to hear: "You do not need to be here. You are handling this in the most incredible way I can possibly imagine, and at this point in time you do not need help."

From my own coping strategies and positive attitude, plus those gleaned from the other caregivers we interviewed, this book was created.

When the Big One Strikes

Michael's diabetes crept up on us, as is often the case with chronic illness. And yet, as is also often the case, we were not totally unaware of what was happening. We had five years of warning signals, annual physicals at which doctors strongly recommended that he cut out smoking and give up sweets. The stubborn strength that made Michael so successful as a corporate negotiator made him sure that he could beat the odds with diabetes, too. We simply failed to realize—or face—the seriousness of the situation.

Chronic illnesses themselves are often difficult to pin down. Sometimes the diagnosis is long in coming, as doctors gradually rule out other possibilities. Many of the people we interviewed for this book knew there was something wrong months, or even years, before a diagnosis was made.

Often, in the initial stages, the caregiver denies what is happening. What the problem is *and that it is forever* simply do not sink in. Connie Hill, an Atlanta psychologist who counsels the families of people with Alzheimer's disease, explains:

> It's not necessarily overt denial. People don't say, "I don't believe this is Alzheimer's disease. It's something else, and I'm not going to try to deal with it." Most of the time it's a more covert type of denial, a refusal or inability to handle any type of education that's there for them, a refusal or inability to take safety precautions with the patient.

Sooner or later, however, there comes a moment when almost every care-giving spouse recognizes that the situation is real and that it is serious. Then there comes a moment when the caregiver internalizes the fact that it is forever, that there is no going back, that life will never be the way it was before the illness came. I recognized the seriousness of Michael's situation when he could no longer walk the beach at Cayman because he was experiencing shooting pains and swelling in his legs. A simple cut on his foot would not heal. Eighteen months and several emergency operations later, he lost a leg, and that was when I realized that the illness was forever.

When the onset of the condition is sudden, both realizations—the seriousness and the Foreverness—often come at once and are accompanied by much activity and confusion. "There is so much going on in the first twenty-four hours that you don't even know what you've done or who's done what," says Joyce, whose husband underwent minor, routine surgery only to have the surgeon stumble upon a malignant tumor nearby. She was forced to come to grips with her status as caregiver to a newly dependent spouse at a time when there was no opportunity for either panic or tears.

Sometimes the caregiver first comes face to face with the irreversibility of a chronic illness the way I did, when the husband or wife comes home from the hospital in a wheelchair or hooked up to an oxygen tank or bedridden. At that point, just the logistical problems that go with getting the person settled in the new situation are enough to take up all your time, not to mention the possibility of having to answer dozens of phone calls from concerned relatives and friends. Everything is focused on the patient, and the caregiver's feelings get pushed aside.

A Jumble of Feelings

The feelings that come with realizing that this situation is forever are always strong and should be dealt with. At forty Irene became the caregiver for her diabetic husband:

> I felt absolute horror at the thought of an "invalid." All of a sudden it hits you that here is this person to be cared for. You think, "I don't want to do that, I can't do that, I'm not going to do that. I'm young, I'm attractive, I've got a life to live. Dear Lord, *you* do it. I'm not doing this." And so you cry for about three days. Then you go out driving on the highway and you listen to all the old songs on the radio and think, "Well, I guess I've got to go home sometime." And then you do.

A person who becomes chronically ill experiences a period of grieving. "When there is a loss through illness," says Dr. Kitty Stein, a psychologist who counsels people with multiple sclerosis, "it feels a lot like a death. Some people call it chronic sorrow, chronic mourning." A chronically ill patient grieves for lost health and for the life he or she formerly led.

The caregiver experiences a similar sense of loss and

goes through a grieving process as well. Often the caregiver's losses mirror those of the patient: freedom and independence, a career or educational program, the opportunity for sexuality, time alone. The caregiver also has to give up the spouse as he or she previously existed and the marriage relationship as it was. From now on everything will be different, because chronic illness affects every facet of the caregiver's life.

When you first learn that your spouse is chronically ill and that you are now a caregiver, some of the feelings you experience will probably shock you. They may be feelings you think are shameful and unworthy, feelings you can never admit to anybody else. Your spouse may never be able to move about without a wheelchair again, breathe without oxygen, or be free of pain and suffering—and yet you feel sorry for yourself, trapped, helpless. You may worry about what's going to happen to your career, or perhaps you are furious at your mate for inflicting his or her condition upon you.

Acknowledge these feelings; they are perfectly normal. I kept a private notebook in which I wrote all my negative feelings. It wasn't a diary or something I felt I had to write in every day about what I had felt or done that day. I called it "Private Moments," and it was the place where I recorded feelings that I thought were important but that I didn't think I could share with anybody. You can't call your confidant or friend every time you hurt. Once I acknowledged to myself a particular feeling or thought I was ashamed of, I'd write it down. It was safe and nonjudgmental. After I wrote it down, I would begin to feel better. My private notebook was an enormous help to me.

Just as it is acceptable for the patient to get angry about his or her lot in life, it is acceptable for the caregiver to get angry also. I usually let Michael know when I was angry and frustrated at his condition and the limitations it placed on my life. (Notice that I was angry at Michael's *condition* but never, never at him for having it. It is important to keep this distinction always in mind.) I sometimes wondered, when I showed my anger in front of Michael, if it was the right thing to do. I was relieved when Dr. Stein confirmed my judgment. "It gives the person who's ill some dignity to feel that someone can get angry with them," she explained. "They're not being treated with kid gloves; they're being treated with dignity."

Try to remember that there were times when you didn't like your mate even when he or she was well—there are in any normal relationship. There will still be times like that, but there's no need to feel guilty about them now just because your mate is chronically ill.

And whatever you do, don't blame yourself for your mate's condition. You are not responsible. Avoid the If Onlys: "If only I had been more adamant that he quit smoking . . ."; "If only I had insisted that she take my car with the good tires when she had to drive in the rain . . ."; and the worst one of all, "If only I had loved him more."

When I found myself being bogged down amid the If Onlys, I told myself that what's past is past and resolved that in the future if I wanted to say something to someone or do something for someone, I would say it or do it at the time. I have been true to my vow on that.

Mental-health professionals teach us that this kind of open communication is important for anybody, sick or well, but it is especially vital in crisis situations such as chronic illness. I found, for example, that I could not always reassure Michael when he was frustrated or afraid. Sometimes when he said, "I'm frightened," I looked him in the eye and said, "I'm frightened, too." Then we could cry together and go forward with a new understanding. I was no longer the stoic tower of false strength with a veil of confidence that nothing could penetrate. I learned to let down my guard, and the resultant honesty opened up a new level of communication for us.

Reach for Help

Of all the emotions I experienced, self-pity was the most

insidious. It would sneak up on me without my being aware of it, tempting me to dwell on Poor Me thoughts. I felt like I was sinking in quicksand. When that happened, I got some kind of help—called up a friend, took a short trip, went to a movie, or even just went out for a walk. That way, I always felt I had a rope within my reach to pull myself up before the quicksand got too deep.

I would advise people who can't find a rope to pull themselves up out of the quicksand, or who realize that they are remaining sad for long periods of time and seeing life as being gray and colorless forever, to seek outside help immediately. *Needing help is nothing to be ashamed of. Not going for it when you know you need it is.* Remember that as a caregiver it is essential to take care of both your mental and your physical health, not only for yourself but for the mate who depends on you.

Chronic illness is an enormous financial drain in many instances and often leaves little money for anything else. If you cannot afford the hourly fees charged by psychologists or psychiatrists in private practice, there is low-cost or no-cost counseling available through state or county mental-health facilities or community crisis centers. Do not be ashamed or afraid to avail yourself of it. It is there for people who need help and can't stretch their budgets any further. Church counselors, ministers, rabbis, and priests are another source of assistance and are experienced in dealing with persons in emotional crisis.

Sometimes the help you need may be as simple as a long talk with a close friend or the opportunity to be alone for a little while. Whether it's an hour of psychiatric counseling or a walk in the park, the objective is always the same: to regain your own self-image and to keep from getting so totally wrapped up in the pain and suffering of your loved one that you come to believe you have no life apart from that.

If the patient's condition warrants it, there are times when you can—and should—go to your mate for help. According to Dr. Stein, "The sick person often feels he or she is the only one in need. If they learn of someone else's needs, then they might be able to help in some way in the problem-solving effort, to get the other person's needs taken care of."

If there was something I wanted very much to do but would take time away from Michael, I always shared it with him, told him why I wanted to do it and how much it meant to me. For example, I said, "I really want to take this volunteer position as president of the Leukemia Society. I know it's going to take time away from you, but this position of leadership is something that means a lot to me and something I really want to contribute." Then I got an agreement from him that he wanted me to go ahead because it was important for me. It was something he could do for me, and giving it to me gave him an additional opportunity to function with dignity.

Form a Support Group

There's safety in numbers, as the saying goes. There's also emotional support. It is always helpful to compare notes with someone in a situation similar to yours. That's a big reason why people in the same kinds of businesses form professional associations, or why students taking the same class will form a study group after school. That's why there are specific support groups for people suffering from cancer, diabetes, lupus, arthritis, head injuries, and a number of other health problems. Alcoholics Anonymous has recognized the importance of support groups for spouses with the formation of Al-Anon for husbands and wives of alcoholics. There are support groups for caregivers of Alzheimer's victims. As far as I know, however, there exists no national network of support groups targeted generally to caregivers of the chronically ill.

That means that if you want one—and I recommend support groups highly—it's up to you to start your own. It shouldn't be too difficult. Start by asking your spouse's doctor or the public-relations director of your hospital for the names and telephone numbers of five people who are in a situation similar to yours—caregivers for mates who are chronically ill. You can confine your search to caregivers for persons suffering from the same disease or form a group for caregivers in general. Call the names on your list and arrange a meeting. If you're afraid to approach a stranger, remember that he or she is probably feeling most of the same feelings you are and would welcome an opportunity to share them with someone else who is in a position to understand—someone like you.

If it is impossible to get away often enough to go to meetings, consider forming a telephone support group. Arrange to phone each other on a regular basis or when you need advice or emotional support. Either way, whether you meet or phone, a support group can be the start of lasting friendships and a strong anchor in times of storm. More than once I called the psychiatrist in New York just to talk and seek advice, because I had no support group.

Getting Back to a New Normal

When I went back to our house after determining I would bring Michael home from the hospital, first I panicked, then I cried—and then I took out my notebook and started taking stock of my situation. Once you've realized that from now on you are going to be your spouse's caregiver, once you have passed through that first panic, and your tears—for the moment at least—are all cried out, you must *assess your situation and determine how you and your family are going to function from this point forward.*

Get a second notebook in addition to the one you keep as a private record of your thoughts. In this one draw up an action plan. First, ask yourself every question you can think of pertaining to your spouse's illness and the impact it will have on your family life. Is the illness truly forever? Is your mate's life span shortened? What will happen if your mate gets worse? Is he or she bedridden? Ambulatory? How does this affect the way you will live?

Walk through an average day. What will you have to do for your spouse during that day? What can he or she do alone? What and how are you going to tell the children? Other relatives? The list will go on and on—but you get the idea. Write down the questions, and answer as many as you have answers for.

Make it a point to learn everything you can about your mate's illness. Ask your doctor for information. Contact the local chapter of the association that represents your spouse's illness if there is one. Haunt the library. Check out books on the illness and on chronic illness in general, as well as books on home health care and adaptive living. Such information will not only help you understand what your mate is going through and what you can expect, but it will stand you in good stead in your relationships with doctors, hospitals, nurses, and other health practitioners as you care for your mate.

Make a list of tasks that have to be done in an ordinary day, once a week, once a month, and once a year. Then figure out how each one will get done. Can you do it? Can your spouse? Can a child? A neighbor or friend? Will you have to hire someone? How much will that cost? Make out an economic plan. What changes in your life-style will have to be made in order to fulfill it?

What you are doing is taking control and establishing a New Normal. Neither your life nor that of your family is going to be the way it was before, but all of you can—and should— become normal again. The only catch is that normal is going to be different than it was before. It is important to establish these new routines as soon as possible, particu- larly when there are children involved. If children know what to expect as best as possible from day to day, then they will have less to fear from the unknown. So will your mate. And so will you. With a feeling of control, you reduce stress and can cope with the long haul.

About the Rest of This Book

That's the beginning. The rest of this book is about the long haul. It discusses what your mate is feeling, how chronic illness changes the balance of a marriage, and the effect that all of this will have on the children—how they feel and how they can be reassured when one of their parents is chronically ill. It suggests how to help friends and relatives understand your situation and how they can be a support system that makes all the difference in your quality of life. It confronts the question of sexuality—how to maintain it and what to do if you can't. It talks about fun times—travel, vacations, hobbies—and how to keep your own spirits up from day to day. It tells how to deal with changes, *how your attitude makes all the difference no matter what occurs*, and how you and your mate can look toward the future with hope. This book also deals with the practical aspects of chronic illness—doctors, hospitals, home care, rehabilitation, other care options, and costs. Finally, there is a chapter on what to do if your spouse does not have long to live.

This is your book. It is designed specifically to answer your questions and concerns as caregiver to a mate who is chronically ill. It is a labor of love that I truly believe will help you.

Bear in Mind:

Recognize that your intense feelings are perfectly normal. A period of grieving is not unusual for a chronically ill person to experience—grief for the life he or she formerly led. The caregiving spouse goes through a similar grieving period.

Find help if you need it. Needing help is nothing to be ashamed of. Not going for it when you know you need it is. As a caregiver, it is essential that you take care of both your mental and physical health, not only for yourself but for the spouse who is depending on you.

Learn everything you can about your mate's illness. It's one way of taking control.

Get back to normal as soon as possible, once your mate's illness has been diagnosed and treatment prescribed. Draw up a list of tasks and assign them among the family. Establish new routines, a New Normal.

2
The Shifting
Marital Balance

M ichael and I were a two-career couple. Part of the strong attraction we had for one another was due to our independence and to the respect each of us had for the other's career and achievements. He was fifty-five and I was forty. We had both been married before, and at this time in our lives we were perfectly content to settle for love and friendship without making our relationship official.

We went along quite happily for two years, and then one sunny day, as we basked in an idyllic beach setting in Grand Cayman, the subject of marriage came up. We talked around it for a while, and then Michael got up the courage to propose. "I don't know," I said. "I'll have to think about it." I spent the next four days putting my thoughts, dreams, and fears down on paper, a process that has always helped me make decisions.

I made a list of questions for Michael, probing questions concerning how he felt about the things that were most important to both of us. Many related to my career, and many related to our children—my two and his four. He answered all of my questions, and I his, to our mutual satisfaction and excitement. Even so, we teased about marrying for "just a year, with an option to renew." In essence we were defining the unwritten rules of the marriage that took place a few weeks later.

Michael was robust and active. Not even in the privacy of my own mind did I think about the possibility of a long-term illness or wonder how it might affect our lives together. But even while we honeymooned in California, a time bomb called diabetes ticked away in Michael's body. Less than four years after our wedding it began disrupting the very fabric of our marriage, putting enormous stresses on our emotions, our life-style, and our careers.

A healthy marriage is a partnership. After the initial courtship phase, you settle in and develop your unspoken roles—the responsibilities, routines, and degree of dependence upon or independence from one another. A balance is worked out that gives a rhythm to your lives: I feed the dog, you take out the garbage; you pay the mortgage, I cover the cost of vacations; I go out occasionally just because I want to, you play cards with the guys at the club with no questions about "who won."

When your partner becomes ill or disabled, this balance changes dramatically. Age is not a factor. It can happen when you are in your twenties, forties, or sixties. The change is unplanned and uninvited, and it permeates every facet of your lives together. The carefully cultivated balance is destroyed, emotions are apt to overrule reason, and everything seems out of control.

From the ensuing chaos emerge new, important issues: What will the future bring? What happens to our careers? Who supports us from now on? How can we afford all this? Who keeps the house in order? How do we deal with all of these losses? *All of these questions must be dealt with before your marriage can find its new balance, its New Normal.*

Living with Not Knowing

One of the realities of chronic illness or disability, whatever the name or cause, is that the future will be uncertain. From now on, you must adjust to living with not knowing. Not knowing whether to buy a one-level house so that your spouse can have maximum mobility. Not knowing whether to cash in your IRA and sell every bit of stock or securities you own in order to be liquid for the forthcoming medical bills. Not knowing whether to accept a promotion or jump at a new business opportunity. Not knowing whether your spouse is going to get substantially worse, stay as is, or go into a period of remission.

Simon's situation illustrates a worst-case scenario of living with not knowing:

> I'd come home at lunchtime, not knowing whether I was going to find Claire watching TV and acting normal, find her having a seizure, or find her dead. Coming home from work, getting up in the morning—I never knew what I might face. So three times a day I held my breath while I looked for my wife. And then I'd get a momentary relief when she was OK. But I never knew what to expect. Try doing that for a couple of months.

Michael and I had been married seven years and had renewed our marital option many times (sometimes once a year, but more recently every few months because of his continuing saga of crisis), when this living with not knowing hit me hardest. Its target was my career.

As an entrepreneur, I create and build businesses. When Michael's illness began, I was totally involved in the largest endeavor I had ever attempted and was already two years into the research and development phase of the project. In most business start-ups the development phase takes more time than planned, and the money runs out long before you believed possible. Desperately in need of advice and interim money, I flew to Chicago to meet with my business mentor. He convinced me that I needed to shift directions and look for a major partner, a move that would take time, energy, and more money—in other words, a consuming commitment on my part. A couple of years before, this wouldn't have been a problem, but now I had a sick husband to consider.

During the meeting I removed my emotional self from

the discussion in order to be rational and use clear, objective thinking. "I'll deal with the emotional side later," I told myself, but it wasn't that easy. A major decision confronted me, and I didn't know whether I should move forward, scale back, or close down and give up. For the first time, I felt the full weight of the past two years of trauma; I found my husband's illness in direct conflict with my own personal and professional dreams. My world was hanging by a thread.

I spent a week examining all of my business options and then made the heartbreaking decision to put a hold on all operations and marketing efforts. When that complex task was done, it was time to tackle the emotions born of worry, disappointment, and pain. I had been suppressing them for a long, long time.

The forty-eighth year of my life is one that continues to haunt me. My mother's Alzheimer's disease took a turn for the worse. After two years of struggle and five operations, Michael lost his left leg to diabetes. Two of our children left home to start their own lives. And my exciting business venture, which for two years had consumed my attention, energy, and drive, came to a sudden and perhaps permanent halt.

Together Michael and I ran away to our house in Grand Cayman, to rest and attempt to regain our perspective on life. Three days into this retreat, just as I was beginning to feel better, I learned that my twelve-year-old dog had died. That was clearly the last straw. I think I cried for a week, the tears of grief going far past the immediate issue and becoming symbolic of everything else I was grieving for: Michael's health, our marriage as it had been, my career, my freedom.

When my tears had dried, it was time to rebuild.

Treading Water

Chronic illnesses come in many forms. Some, like diabetes and multiple sclerosis, are slow and degenerative. Some, like heart attacks, are sudden and acute, and you don't know if the loved one will survive the first few days. Some don't make their existence known until a routine exam uncovers something that sends everyone into a state of shock. Whatever the scenario, *the surviving spouse must take control as soon as possible after the initial blow and make a temporary plan.*

People who have suffered a major shock—such as the death of a loved one—are often advised to make no major decisions for at least a year. Chronic illness can be just as disruptive as a death and should be treated accordingly. When my new business venture was suspended, I was strongly advised not to try to force a solution. I made an informal commitment to myself to postpone any major decisions for at least six months or until I knew what was going to happen with Michael's health. As a result, however, I found myself unmotivated, unfulfilled, and bored. I felt like I was treading water.

I, who had always been goal oriented, had no goals now. Instead, I was keeping my eyes, ears, and mind open for a sign, a word, a direction. This transition time was purposeful, I soon realized, because it gave me a chance to refocus, to find out what the New Normal in my business life would be.

Vanessa, a writer, also experienced this. She was pregnant when her husband had a cerebral aneurysm that left him permanently disabled:

> I had already planned to scale back for three months because of the baby. Fortunately, I was self-employed. If I'd had a regular job, I probably would have lost it because this interim time period lasted over eight months. A benevolent company will give you several months' disability leave if you are in the executive ranks, but there are many people who are not so fortunate.

Vanessa's method of taking control was to find freelance writing that was noncreative, close to home, and part time.

Her part-time work paid for a housekeeper and helped her maintain a grasp on reality. "For a long time I just treaded water while I refocused," she says.

Treading water is a survival method. If the boat sinks and you can't swim the distance to shore, treading water allows you to remain afloat until help comes along. Once I had treaded water long enough to get my bearings, I began addressing my dilemma. After putting my new venture on hold, I delayed my previous plans to move to a new, modern office complex. Instead we moved to a smaller office— right next door so our company could keep the same telephone number and address. I utilized freelance people to fulfill existing obligations, and I hired temporaries for secretarial work.

Work: The Justifiable Escape

This phase lasted about eighteen months and was essentially a nonproductive time. Why, then, did I keep on working? *I did it as much for Michael as for myself, because I believed I must remain the same person he had married.* He didn't really want me to change, because I got much of my energy and vitality from the outside world. If I went out and got "pumped up," I could continue to take care of him.

I also worked to keep my balance, another important factor if I was to give Michael the best of myself. If I had stayed home I could have become bitter and angry, and in such a negative state I wouldn't have had much to offer anyone, much less a sick and cranky husband. Dr. Jeanne Shaw, a clinical psychologist, helps to explain:

> It's always better for the dependent person to be angry with the caretaker than it is for the caretaker to be angry with the dependent person, because the dependent person's survival depends on the good will of the person taking care of him or her. They have to strike a balance with one another. The care/sacrifice/ treatment should be appropriate for the wound: if somebody's bone is sticking through the skin, you're not going to say, "I have to go to the office." But if

your partner is depressed and irritable, you don't stay home just to try to cheer them up.

Don't massage their dependency needs. Only take care of the physical necessities that the other person literally cannot take care of himself. Shelly Cox, the author of *If You Meet Buddha on the Road—Kill Him*, says that whenever you do something for people that they could do for themselves, you have diminished them in some way. We tend to diminish disabled people by thinking they can't do things for themselves, physically and mentally. In other words, do not protect them from things that might be unpleasant for them.

Frank, a cancer patient, agrees. During his worst crisis he wanted only to be cared for, and he thinks it would have been easy to remain in that helpless mode had his wife Ann given in to his demands:

> When you are wiped out in the hospital, you expect other people to take care of you. But when you're out of that environment and back in the real world, you've got to start getting off your rear end if you're going to make it. My wife pushed me a lot. I didn't want to get out and walk. But just like she pushed me in the hospital to sit in the chair and play games to get my mind going again, when I got home she pushed me to walk. To walk two or three blocks would take me thirty or forty minutes, but in the end it paid off.

Ann got Frank back on his feet just enough to free her for a return to work. "I offered to quit two or three times," she says, "but I didn't, I think because I wasn't being pressured to, and because my employer valued me. That felt good."

I, too, needed to enhance my self-image, which was becoming battered from all the changes, rebalancing, and new roles. Being valued by people out there in the real world, away from the needy person at home, was vital to my self-esteem. Most of us also view work as an escape from the relentless pressure at home. "Working was a salvation for me," says one female executive, "because I could get somewhere and make decisions without feeling like I was walking on eggshells, the way I did at home."

No More Show-and-Tell

Chronic illness brings with it many losses. One of the saddest is the personality transformation of the person you chose to share your life with. Vicki and Brad have been married twenty-three years. Vicki was and still is an executive for a well-known, medium-size company, on the fast track toward an impressively outstanding career. Brad was the distinguished senior executive of a major corporation when heart disease ended his career. He has had three coronaries, two pacemakers, and triple-bypass surgery. He takes medication that would affect the mental, emotional, and marital balance of any relationship. Because he has not worked since his first heart attack twelve years ago, Vicki has no one at home to share her successes with:

> The first ten years of our marriage it was show-and-tell. We would come home in the afternoon and be full of ourselves, telling what we did, what we said, who we saw, or how we won a sale. Then suddenly there was no more show-and-tell on his part. I had to stop sharing my day with Brad because he didn't want to hear about these wonderful things.

Brad is now capable of participating in his own events and activities but chooses not to, and he consequently has a feeling of being a noncontributor. Vicki deals with this by studying the characteristics of his personality and the illness that he has. Even though she continues to balance her own needs with his, Brad has become resentful of the time her work and civic activities take away from him. "We tried to talk about it," she says, "but he makes such a mountain out of a molehill that it's almost impossible."

But shoveling the problem under the carpet doesn't help

anyone. It is important to discuss your expectations of each other, and the ones that are no longer possible need to be explored and redefined. *If some of the expectations and realities are no longer possible, then you must accept them as a loss and grieve.*

Vanessa and Dennis had been married nine years before his aneurysm left him brain-damaged—perhaps the most devastating type of loss of all. Vanessa has lost the person she married, yet she still lives with him:

> This was my best friend in all the world—my soul-mate. I lost my intellectual companion. Dennis was incredibly bright, but after the aneurysm his thinking processes were impaired. I still love him, but I look on him with sorrow. What is a mind? What is character? What is personality? If these things are damaged in brain trauma, everything is altered.
>
> We loved each other and had a very good marriage. He was the perfect man for me. I still love him dearly, and that is the thing that makes me go home each night. But when I see a healthy man—even just a strong biceps in an elevator—I feel wistful. I know everything has changed, and it makes me sad. I know that I am never going to have that again.

But Vanessa has been able to grieve for her loss and consequently to let go a little:

> I've reconciled myself to the notion that these periods of sadness are normal. They don't mean I'm crazy; they don't mean I'm not coping well. They're a realistic and appropriate response to a profound tragedy in someone's life. I'm perfectly justified in feeling sad. To do otherwise would be trying to deny it. I've come to accept that I'm going to go through these stages.
>
> There was a point at which I let go. I realized that I couldn't rely on Dennis for emotional support, for analytical assistance, for physical assistance day to day—for anything. And that's a real shocker to come to with your spouse. What are you going to do about that? You're either going to collapse in a puddle, or

you're going to pick yourself up and say, "If he can't do it, I'm going to do it."

Grieving for things lost is necessary before you can begin to get your marriage in balance again. Perhaps that is what I was doing when, after aborting my new business venture, I ran away and cried for a week. I was grieving that my husband was no longer the person I married and that the prestige and momentum of my own career were shattered. I felt as if I had lost my own identity and was no longer in control of my own destiny.

New Roles, New Demands

In any marriage, the various responsibilities are shared by two people. When one half of the team is down, the other must shoulder the full burden—in addition to caring for the sick one. This can triple the workload. As one female caregiver put it, "It's like being a widow without the benefits."

First comes a need for organization, a time-consuming task for a busy person who already has too many burdens to bear. For someone like Vicki who was immersed in her work, it was hard to find the time for attending to all of these extra details:

> Extraordinary demands were placed on me to provide physical care, find resources, find contacts, find employees for when I could not be there. Twelve years ago that was pretty hard to do; at our young ages, we didn't have the resources built in. I had to learn file-building and management skills for my personal life as well as for my business life, because one-half of this team had been effectively eliminated from routine activity. Who mows the lawn every Saturday, who puts the roof on the house, who does all those chores that one-half of the team had managed?

"What I needed through all of this was a wife," she adds, a strange but appropriate statement from a woman who

found playing the roles of both husband and wife an almost overwhelming task.

Complicating the need for organization is the financial adjustment required by medical bills, loss of income, or both. One husband, whose wife had Alzheimer's diagnosed at the very young age of fifty-three, had to say good-bye to the dreams he had harbored during years of hard work. "It was a great disappointment," he says. "Our youngest child had one more year of college and then we expected to be free and do some traveling. All our plans went up in smoke."

The new responsibilities heaped upon the caregiver can vary according to sex. For a man, the added responsibilities are primarily on the domestic front; he must take on the household chores his wife formerly handled:

> I've had to pick up a lot of the household duties; I've had to organize my time very closely. That's probably the biggest adjustment, the time that I have to spend doing things that I would not formerly have done— laundry, house cleaning, and occasional meal preparation—all the things our wives normally have to do on top of their own jobs!

For a woman, on the other hand, the most frightening aspect of becoming head of the household can be the shouldering of the entire financial burden. Vanessa was shocked by the weight of the responsibility she had to assume when her husband was no longer able to work:

> *I had to start thinking like a man.* Please understand how difficult that was for me. I grew up with the women's movement, *Ms.* magazine, and independence, but I was kidding myself with what I thought I knew. I had to start thinking like a man—to have a career to support my husband, my child . . . to support a family!

Vanessa and Dennis have experienced a complete role

reversal. She has shouldered the full burden of earning a living while he takes up the slack on the household front, although the major home management still falls on her since Dennis has lost what she calls his "executive functions."

The Ripple Effect

While the world of the two of you is shifting, adjusting, and seeking to find a New Normal, your actions are affecting numerous other lives around you, both at work and within your family. I will address the family and friends issues later but want to touch on the work issue here.

Because priorities have shifted dramatically, the spreading circle of losses begins to affect the caregiver's work. Many people lose confidence, lose their creativity, or can't focus. I felt an overwhelming amount of organizational frustration, of being pulled in a thousand different directions. When you work, whether for a company or for yourself, it can be a real juggling act to take time off to attend to the myriad details at home without letting your boss or your clients down in the process. Although they are usually understanding and sympathetic, there is still a risk of jeopardizing the job or missing deadlines.

Some people, like me, have to scale back. Others may have to pass up a promotion or transfer, or let go of a personal goal. This happened to Vicki:

> I had an opportunity to run for elective office in government, and when I decided not to run, it felt like a big loss. I feel like I let every woman in the world down. I feel that I had the opportunity to make a bold statement and did not take it. But Brad has had twelve years of life that he had not expected to have, so I have tried to adjust my business life to balance the two.

For some women, plowing ahead with a career can cause

secondary problems. When a man's wife becomes ill, no one expects him to give up his job to stay home and care for her. In fact, friends and relatives are sometimes more eager to help so that he doesn't disrupt his career goals. But when a woman's husband is struck down, society often condemns her for carrying on with her career. This pressure can give her the impression that she is fighting for her very survival as a person.

Polly was in medical school when her husband was diagnosed with a cerebellar tumor. After its surgical removal he hovered on the brink of death for weeks, then was left with permanent disabilities. In the face of family pressure to drop everything and "do her duty," Polly decided to carry on with her plans:

> I'm very selfish; it didn't affect my career plans at all. My family thought I was the worst person in the world, but I continued with what I did. Actually, in some ways that was probably the best thing, because I didn't dwell on Al's illness and hover over him. He was forced to resume primary caregiving of our small child and to continue with his teaching career. Although it wasn't easy, in retrospect I believe that it forced him to get back into the mainstream.

Many women have no choice but to keep working. Women now make up more than 44 percent of the work force in the United States, and two-career couples are the norm. Polly's family didn't stop to consider how she would support herself and her son if Al died—or how much easier their future would be on her doctor's salary.

For Vanessa, Dennis's illness necessitated a complete change in her career goals:

> I was out in the ocean. It was either sink or swim— and I had to start swimming in a different direction as well. I could no longer work at home because my husband and the baby were driving me crazy, so I rented a small office nearby, bought a computer, and

got serious. I learned how to sell, how to do my own bookkeeping accurately, and whatever else it took. In one year I doubled my income, and I tripled it the next. I've held steady since then. Now, for the first time, I can breathe a little easier.

Vanessa is one of the lucky ones whose career blossomed under the added pressure. For some, like me, the career temporarily suffered. And for others, like Jesse, the damage was permanent:

> I would have been more aggressive in my career, but I always thought that any additional responsibility I took on would mean that I had to contribute less at home. While I have a very good job, I accepted certain plateaus in my career that I wouldn't have accepted otherwise.

"Why Do You Have to Work So Much?"

I believe that in marriages where both of the partners have careers and independence, they gather strength from that independence. The Show-and-Tell portion of the day is shared with love and genuine interest. I also feel that even in this generation of accepted two-career couples there is still an area of mixed emotions over the new roles. When illness strikes down one partner, it exacerbates that confusion. In my case, while Michael was genuinely proud and supportive of my career, he was also lonely once he began spending most of his life at home. Because he was now dependent on me, he became jealous of anything that ate into our time together.

During the first year or two of his plight, this resentment was expressed in subtle ways. Part of my style of doing business is to develop contacts and build relationships, often socially over lunch or dinner. This was one of the issues we had discussed before we were married, and at that time it had posed no problem. Now that Michael was sick, though, he didn't feel quite the same about my need for "relationship selling" because instead of being busy with his own interests while I was away, he was sitting at home impatiently awaiting my return. He might greet my arrival with a comment like, "What could you possibly have talked about for so long?" or with an innuendo about the uselessness of my volunteer work. Although he knew my strong feelings about not ever wanting to work from a home office again, he periodically suggested that I do just that, especially once I began scaling down my operations. To me, doing that would have been equivalent to tossing away my life raft even while my ship was taking on water. It was a great pull, and the unpleasantness of it often made coming home difficult. But I resisted his subtle pressure and let my survival instincts continue to guide me.

Many two-career marriages experience vacillations in emotions regardless of the health of the partners. It seems to be human nature to become envious and possessive when work takes on more importance than the primary relationship. Communication—talking to one another on a "feeling" level—is the quickest way to work through this confusion. It does not guarantee instant success, but it keeps the pipeline open and increases sensitivity until a possible solution is reached.

The Connubial Seesaw

In any relationship, the two partners work together like a couple of kids on a seesaw. When one is down, the other is up, and his weight eventually brings the other up to a higher level. The balance is never fifty/fifty; it is constantly changing. When chronic illness strikes, the patient spends more time on the low end, but just because someone is down most of the time doesn't mean that he can't give an enormous push once in a while and experience again the giddiness that comes from being the one higher in the air.

Nineteen eighty-seven was for me a year of major trauma. During the drabness of that winter Michael spent five weeks in intensive care, fighting for his remaining leg and his life. He lost the battle for the leg, and for a time it appeared that he would lose the larger battle as well. Every system in his body broke down, and the subsequent weeks of caring for him took every bit of strength I possessed.

Then, only a few months later, my mother died, and my world came apart. There was absolutely no reserve left in me. That is when Michael became *my* caregiver. For the next several weeks he took over as head of the household. It was such an astonishing thing to witness that even in the midst of my grief I relished every moment of what was happening. I can only imagine the renewed sense of strength and pride Michael must have felt by being able to repay me for what I had done for him.

He never again lapsed back into his prior state of emotional dependency. He continued to take an aggressive stance in keeping me busy with things outside of work, outside of him. Because we'd had to sell our house on Grand Cayman, we came up with the idea of getting a place on Lake Lanier, thirty miles out of Atlanta, and he was the one who pushed me to keep looking until we were eventually led to the place I now call home. The setting was so peaceful, so pregnant with new life and hope, that instead of buying a weekend cabin we bought a large house and moved in permanently. Decorating, and making the changes needed for Michael and his wheelchair, kept us both busy for months and kept us outside of ourselves and our immediate problems. After months of remaining stationary and unbalanced, the seesaw had again tipped. When it did, it brought our entire marital balance to a new level of love and caring.

BEAR IN MIND:

Continue to work as much for your spouse as for yourself.

Accept the limitations. If some of the expectations and realities are no longer possible, then you must accept them as a loss and grieve.

If you are a woman, do not be afraid to continue your career. When a man's wife becomes ill, no one expects him to give up his job in order to stay home and care for her. But when a woman's husband is struck down, society sometimes condemns her for carrying on with her career.

Allow your spouse to become your caregiver. Imagine the renewed sense of strength and pride he or she must feel by being able to repay you for what you have done.

3
From the Patient's Point of View

"You have no idea what it's like," the patient tells the caregiver plaintively. In truth, the caregiver does not. In Ernest Hemingway's "In Another Country," a short story about wounded soldiers receiving treatment at a hospital in Milan, the word "country" does not refer only to Italy. It alludes to a foreign land where there are no road maps or signposts and where the language is indecipherable. The patient explores it alone. The caregiver might listen to stories and read books about that strange country, but he or she cannot visit it to share the experience.

It is no wonder that such a lonely exploration affects the patient's personality. Some facets are enhanced, others recede, and after a time the patient is no longer the same person as before. There is, however, an understandable tendency on the caregiver's part to respond as though this were not so, as though the patient is the same as ever. Because we ourselves do not personally experience the pain, fear, and guilt the patient is going through, we have difficulty accepting the changes these create in his or her former personality.

Alone on Another Planet

For the one who is sick, a sense of isolation prevails. Arthur, who is terminally ill, explains why:

No one else understands. People can try. The person who probably comes closest to understanding the frustration is my mother, who watched my father die of this and now is seeing me go through the same thing. But there is a line: if you're on one side you deal with it, if you're on the other side you're an observer. You can be a very good observer, you can have it explained to you, but it is impossible to accurately feel another person's emotions.

Beth suffered for eight years from a rare and serious allergic condition that left her dizzy, weak, and sick:

Looking back now, it felt like being on another planet with a blinding white sky, sand that burned under my feet, and a wind always blowing hot against me. There was no water, no shade, and nothing in the distance, not even a mirage. I was alone there, with no one to comfort me.

Beth's new and rare disease, which is currently being called Ecological Illness, involves a breakdown in the immune system. She has become what is known as a "universal reactor," meaning that she is allergic to almost everything. For eight years she was virtually a prisoner in her own house, as vivid an example of emotional isolation as one can imagine:

Because my illness was so bizarre, a lot of people thought I was crazy. Some thought I had agoraphobia—that I was afraid of leaving my own house. Anorexia was another thing people could suspect me of having, because there were so few foods I could digest, I was down to ninety-five pounds. It made me very paranoid, because I never knew who thought I was crazy and who didn't.

Even Beth's husband, George, became a little suspicious of her. Fortunately, one particularly astute doctor insisted that George come along to an allergy demonstration. When the offending substances were applied to Beth's skin, George witnessed firsthand the dizziness and mental confusion they provoked, and the subsequent disappearance of those symptoms when the substances were removed. For the first time he could clearly see that his wife had a medical problem, not a psychiatric one. This was a great help, but didn't solve everything. According to Beth, "George admitted at one point that he had some paranoia about whether I had just married him because I knew this was going to happen and needed somebody to take care of me." Talk about emotional isolation!

Contributing to this isolation is the consuming nature of illness. *Chronic illness is like a strangler vine, entwining itself around every thought and every action, threatening to suffocate the very soul.* If your spouse was formerly the type to keep silent about minor illnesses, he or she may now refuse to discuss this major one and will withdraw into a private world of suffering. If, in contrast, he or she used to keep you informed of small complaints, you can expect to be kept abreast of major ones as well—perhaps more abreast than you would like. Because life now revolves around the discomfort, the disabilities, the drugs, and the fear, the patient's attention zeros in on each new symptom and what it might mean. It becomes so consuming that the caregiver soon grows weary of hearing about it. Beth and George had to make a pact to help keep things under control:

> I agreed to share only those details of my illness that affected him. We chose a place in the dining room where I would take him every day when he came home from work and tell him everything I thought he needed to know. We also imposed a time limit on these conversations. We simply had to contain this thing.

Whether your spouse attempts to share more than you are willing to hear, or whether he or she withdraws, emotional isolation is a factor you must be aware of so you can keep the channels of communication open and the distance between the two of you as narrow as possible.

Living in Fear

Fear is another contributor to changes in personality. Fear makes the ill person timid, reticent, tentative—or else a sudden daredevil, bent on proving that nothing has changed. And fear runs rampant when one's own body becomes a traitor. What is there left to trust? Each new symptom brings fresh terror, and until its implications are understood, the heart thumps, the adrenaline flows, and the emotional reaction can be all out of proportion to the seriousness of each individual event. Beth had a particularly hard time:

> Because I was a universal reactor, I became afraid of everything. Windy days. Pollen from oak trees. Insecticide. Mold in heating systems. I could tell when the heat came on in a large office building or at the airport because it made me dizzy.

If the illness strikes suddenly, the immediate and crushing fear almost takes one's breath away. When the diagnosis comes after years of worrying about a variety of symptoms that have been misdiagnosed, the fear is more insidious. At first there might be a flood of relief that people will at last believe in the existence of real illness, that there will be no more insinuations of psychiatric problems, but the relief is followed shortly thereafter by horror at the diagnosis and its sentence of permanent disability. Cynthia struggled to accept the verdict of lupus that was laid over her like a shroud of impending doom:

> My biggest problem was actually accepting the fact that I was sicker than I had ever been before. This time it wasn't just another one of those weird ill-

nesses that I'd had in the past; this time they said it wasn't ever going to go away. That was a big emotional insult. I was scared to death.

So was Beth, struggling with Ecological Illness that no one seemed to know much about. "For three years I was scared at every moment of every day that I was going to die," she can now admit. In addition, she had to struggle with anxiety that was of clinical origin, one of the manifestations of her allergies. This brought about yet another worry:

> I had a fear of losing control, of being in a business situation when the heat came on or when somebody came through with Windex to clean something. If even minute amounts of the substances I reacted to were in the air, my muscles got weak, I couldn't concentrate, and I got anxious. I was afraid that a client might see me do that.

Fear undermined Michael's confidence—and he had been a supremely confident man. His major fear related to me. He felt that he was getting old, no longer able to be my husband in every sense of the word. At the same time I seemed—in his eyes, at least—to be getting "younger, more lovely, and in the prime of [my] life." He was afraid I would leave him. At those times I didn't try to tell him that he shouldn't be feeling that way. I didn't say, "There, there. Don't cry. It will be OK," the way many well-meaning people do when they feel helpless and uncomfortable around someone who is upset. Instead I acknowledged that what he was feeling was real. I then "renewed his option" on our marriage for another three months. This was a joking manner of expressing our continuing love.

Fear of abandonment is not unusual. The sick one worries not only that the caregiver might walk out on the marriage, but that something terrible will happen: a car accident, a heart attack, a plane crash—the possibilities that the imagination calls forth are endless. Being in a constant state of dependency is bad enough, but the thought of having to survive alone is almost beyond comprehension.

Akin to the fear of abandonment is the patient's intuition—or knowledge—that he or she will be the one to leave the family behind. Katy faces this four or five times a year when her asthma sends her to intensive care for yet another fight for life. She encourages her husband to function as independently as possible, even to the point of spending a considerable amount of time working away from home. "If anything ever happened it wouldn't be quite so painful," she says, but I'm not sure I agree. The pain of losing a loved one will not lessen simply because the survivor is independent.

Another fear of Michael's was that his doctors might be withholding information. I unwittingly contributed to this by planning my hospital visits to coincide with the doctors' rounds. That allowed me to have a private moment with them in the hallway when nobody could interrupt. Afterward, when I breezed into Michael's room, he'd say, "Oh, too bad, you just missed the doctor." I would answer, "No, I spoke with the doctor in the hall," not noticing the wary look that passed across his face. Had I been more sensitive I would have brought those conversations into the doorway of Michael's room instead of letting him worry about what the doctor might have said behind his back.

The fear of death—an undeniable accompaniment to most chronic illnesses—is strong in the human race. People will do almost anything to hang on; witness the Holocaust survivors. Most of the people we spoke with who had been informed that their condition was terminal were coping well, perhaps because none was yet close to the end. Most were still in the denial phase, although some had already come to grips with death after many close brushes. Only one or two were in a state of terror that could not be verbalized.

If your spouse is struggling through this type of adjustment, some aspects of the fear can be lessened by talking and reading, by bringing the subject out of the dark corners of the mind and into the light of day (Elisabeth Kübler-Ross's books are a good place to start). Michael claimed not to be afraid of death, but he expressed a concern that he would "wind up rotting in a box in the ground." It was so worrying to him that I encouraged him to add a request for cremation to his will, which he did.

A Constant State of Grief

The losses that the patient experiences go far beyond the issue of health. Cynthia describes the losses she has suffered:

> I had to give up my job. I had to give up my plans to go to medical school. I was dealing with my physical changes. I was dealing with the loss of my health which involves a grief process just like losing a family member does. I was dealing with the loss of my sexuality.
>
> I had to give up the independence that I had always enjoyed in my relationship with my husband: we led very independent life-styles, we had chosen not to have any children, we each had a career. I had never depended on him for money or anything else. Then I became a dependent person, which was a totally new experience because I had never been totally dependent in all of my adult life.

Michael lost his mobility, his freedom, his independence, and the ability to control his own destiny. The last few months of his life he also lost his personal dignity when he couldn't even get from the bed to the bathroom without help. But *perhaps the greatest loss for Michael—even greater than the loss of his legs—was the loss of power.* This must be true for anyone with a career, but it is not a loss that is normally acknowledged. Michael continued to go to the office whenever he could, but because he was away so much of the time, he lost his authority. People no longer came to him for decisions because he was not there often enough for them to do so. Colleagues stopped calling him for his opinion on matters related to business. They might call to tell him what they had done, but they no longer called to ask what he thought they should do. He was no longer a member of the team.

Another loss commonly experienced by the chronically ill is the loss of opportunity. Michael could have become president of his company, but because he was physically incapacitated he was passed over for promotion. All chronically ill people lose opportunities—for new jobs, for promotions, for travel. And many lose something that should be a basic right of all human beings—the chance to have children.

Endless Frustration and Bouts of Rage

The resulting frustration is constant. "There isn't a day that goes by that I'm not somehow aware of my own disabilities," says one patient. Those who are bedridden are bored much of the time. Those with a debilitating illness lack the energy to perform even the simplest household tasks. Those in unremitting pain are worn down by the drain on their will. And those restricted to wheelchairs lack the mobility to go many public places, a hurdle that society has done little to lower. Beth was frustrated because she could no longer work the way she used to:

> I couldn't control my work situation. I couldn't go out and solicit the kind of business I wanted. I had to turn down a position I had waited a year for, because when it opened I was too sick to go and apply for it. There was nothing I could do that was anything like a normal life. Everything frustrated me.

The frustration can lead to deeper feelings of despair. For some, like Hank's wife, depression lurks just around the corner, waiting to rear its ugly head:

When my wife found out she had Alzheimer's she searched for everything she could find about it. Of course the more she read and realized what was going to happen to her, the more depressed she became. She cried an awful lot, and she talked about suicide on half a dozen occasions, feeling that was a better out than having to go through what she knew was coming.

Others are consumed by rage. Sonya describes the anger that her husband Jerry developed after he became paralyzed from a fall:

> His anger was unbelievable. When he was first in his wheelchair he couldn't reach anything, but rather than ask for help he broke everything in sight. He screamed at me, "Get out! Go away!" I answered, "I have no place to go, and I love you."
>
> He was in rehabilitation in one of the best facilities in California; I was at our ranch nine miles away. One day when he was first at the rehab center, it was time to come home, but he had not yet learned to transfer from the wheelchair into the taxicab. He was so angry, and so proud, that he wheeled nine miles home—in the rain. His rage prevented him from calling me.

Michael's growing weakness and dependency often made him lash out, usually at whichever kid was nearest. Fortunately, the one who was around the most during the last year or two could take it. With a wisdom that belied his age, he understood the reasons behind the antagonism, and whatever the subject matter, he rarely debated or argued. Another of Michael's outlets was downright rebellion, almost of the teenage variety. His smoking was a good example, even though smoking played a big part in his illness. His own vascular surgeon once said, "If I ever see you smoking again I'll personally cut off your other leg." And yet Michael would disappear into the bathroom for half an hour, and I'd see smoke curling out from under the door.

A few patients, like Beth, are able to push the destructive feelings aside:

> I was so angry and so frustrated that something just snapped, and I didn't feel much of it anymore. I realized that it was so injurious to my immune system to indulge in those feelings that I just didn't. I don't think I repressed them; in an odd sort of way I simply let them go.

You must always keep in mind that it's not *you* the patient is angry with, it's the situation. When those outbursts occur, a caregiver has several choices of how to react. One is to keep cool and collected as though there is a Plexiglas shield between the two of you. If some arrows manage to pierce it, you can always cry later in privacy. Since I am a nonconfrontive person, this was my typical response, although it had a tendency to backfire because it drives combative personalities (like Michael's) crazy. Another choice is to yell back. If that is your normal behavior, then let loose. There are enough changes occurring in your marriage already without you stifling the personality your husband or wife chose to marry. A third choice would be to pull back far enough to gain a more objective perspective. One caregiver used a technique of saying to himself, "What if the roles were reversed? What would she do for me?"

The Burden of Guilt

So often Michael would ask, "How do you put up with me?" Most dependent people feel guilty about wrecking their loved ones' lives, using up all the family savings, and cutting off most social opportunities and chances for fun. Beth carries a particularly heavy load of guilt because she was struck down only a month after her wedding:

I feel enormously guilty. We had signed a marital contract stipulating that we would each cover 50 percent of the expenses, support each other emotionally, and so on, and I couldn't hold up my end of the contract. We would have a substantially different lifestyle if this hadn't happened.

For a long time I felt awful because we were so poor. The house was falling down, and the furniture was falling apart. It looked terrible, and I was ashamed of it. Everywhere I looked there was something to remind me of our dire poverty and that it was all my fault. I would look at my peers and see the money they were making and the level of jobs they had and the creative types of work they were doing, and I would feel guilty because I couldn't do that. I also feel enormously guilty for the adverse impact that I've had on George's life.

People suffering under a great burden of guilt often try to compensate in some way. Katy says she tries to be a "better-than-good wife," even to the extent of compromising her health by not going to the hospital when she should. Beth compensates by putting extra effort into her work, trying to earn enough money to ease the financial strain on her husband. She has covered all expenses connected with her illness, including the cost of changing the house's heating system from gas to electricity since she's allergic to gas, buying an electric water heater, and installing additional insulation and storm windows. "That was a way to buy my way out of some of my guilt," she admits.

Like the husband or wife who tries to assuage the guilt of a divorce by giving everything to the spouse until hardly enough is left to live on, a patient may sometimes sacrifice too much out of guilt. The care-giving spouse must be aware of this possibility and guard against it, because if the patient gives too much, he or she can become resentful of the care-giving spouse for accepting it. What appeared freely given can have strings attached that go unnoticed by both parties until it's too late.

Guilt can be alleviated by the caregiver's constant reassurance. When Michael asked, "How do you put up with me?" the answer I usually gave was, "It ain't easy, but you do have some redeeming values." I'd mention a few, such as, "You're cute," or "You have enough hair left that I can still run my fingers through it." I tried to lighten things up. He needed enormous reassurance, and I worked very hard at giving it to him.

Who's that Ugly Person in the Mirror?

We once took some family photos in Michael's hospital room. When he saw them, he was appalled. "I look like I'm dead," he said in anguish. Once a positive self-image goes out the window nearly everything else follows, so anything you can do to improve things will be well worth the effort. When Michael became distraught over his appearance, I brought him a sun lamp, and he looked so good after using it for a few weeks that he went out and bought some new suits.

It was not quite that easy after the first amputation. As part of his rehabilitation program he had a masseuse, but after his first amputation a long time went by before he could muster the courage to let her see him again.

Loss of a positive self-image can make a patient reclusive. Michael strongly disliked having to let people know he was back in the hospital again. "Don't tell anyone!" he always pleaded. I suppose he was ashamed that he was once again "failing" and out of control of his own destiny. Of course I had to tell the children, but Michael's pleas sometimes kept me from telling others. After four or five days of sitting in the hospital without a phone call or a visitor or a card he would become quite grumpy, but he could never see that it was his own doing. I learned to deal with the problem by honoring his requests for secrecy for only two or three days. Then, if it looked like this was going to be a long stay, I planted a seed at Michael's office, suggesting nonchalant phone calls or visits rather than cards and flowers. I didn't like to "cry wolf" unless the situation indeed warranted extra concern.

For Katy and many others who are on chronic steroid therapy, oftentimes a self-image problem is drug-related:

> You blow up like a balloon, and your whole body image is changed. That's difficult to cope with in a marriage. When I got terribly ill last year I went from 135 pounds to 165 pounds in about three and a half weeks. It was just awful.

As a person becomes more comfortable with an illness, particularly if it responds to treatment, feelings can pick up considerably. Beth describes how her self-image has evolved over the past eight years:

> At first I saw myself as a sick person. I was even sick in my dreams. As I got better I entered into a stage where I saw myself as a person who was sick most of the time. Then I thought of myself as somebody who was beginning to recover. There were subtle gradients. Now I see myself as someone who may have chronic problems for the rest of my life but can lead a fairly normal existence. I don't see myself as normal, but I see myself as someone who can be mistaken for normal. That solves a lot of problems.

The problems she refers to are those she has with acquaintances and with the public, with people who ask, "How are you?" without really wanting an honest answer.

Katy finds that keeping herself well-groomed helps her self-image considerably while also staving off potentially awkward conversations with some of her more casual acquaintances:

> I can be feeling like hell, but I know how to do my makeup now so that they don't know a thing about what's going on with me personally. Many people keep asking how I feel, but they don't really want to

know; they just want to sound empathetic. I deal with it by just saying, "Fine," except to my very close friends.

But looking too healthy can have a negative side. "People think that you should be unkempt if you are sick," says Katy. "If you don't look sick they think you're malingering." It can be hard to find a balance.

What's Wrong with That Man?

What should be important is how *we* perceive ourselves, not what other people think, but no matter how much we'd like it to be otherwise, public reaction still influences how we feel. "I think I look fine," says one patient, "but every now and then I still run into that individual who reminds me that there's something wrong." Arthur, who carts around an oxygen tank wherever he goes, classifies the public into four groups:

> Children, small children, will go ask their mommies, "What's wrong with that man?" or "What's that man got?" That's easy to put up with, especially since I have a small child myself. Kids have a natural curiosity.
>
> Occasionally people will come up to me because they've had a family member who's had either lung disease or heart disease and has been on oxygen. They'll say, "Gee, it's really nice to see someone who's out doing the things you're doing. My late husband . . ." and try to give me encouragement. That's people trying to be nice, typically older ladies.
>
> There are some people, especially people who know me, who sort of matter-of-factly ask, "What is that?" Very objective. That's easy to deal with. I can say, "It's oxygen, I have it because . . ." Almost an engineering approach.
>
> But there are other people who—I guess when any of us see someone with a deformity, we look but we

don't look. Avert our eyes. "There but for the grace of God," that sort of thing. And I see that quite a bit. That can be annoying at times.

It can be more than just annoying when people are downright rude. Katy, who has a permanent tracheotomy, never ceases grappling with public reaction:

> People can be awfully tactless. Recently I went to a cancer seminar, and during the break a woman at the next table turned around and said, "Have you got laryngitis?" This was a professional group made up of people who treat oncology patients, and there I am with a tracheotomy—which was obvious because I have to put my finger over it to speak. With people who don't know better, I don't feel angry, but people who should know better *do* make me angry. I had a friend with me who said, "I had no idea what it was like, for people who are chronically sick, to put up with that kind of stupid remark on a day-to-day basis."

How do people like Katy respond to such remarks?

> Usually the best way to deal with questions is to be honest. "No, I have a tracheotomy," I say matter-of-factly, because people feel uncomfortable once they know they've made a boo-boo. That can escalate if you don't either joke about it or just tell them how it is: "No, I have a chronic respiratory condition, and I will never talk properly." They feel more relaxed that you can tell them.

Allen, who is a teacher, has residual effects from the surgical removal of a brain tumor. He uses his disabilities as a teaching tool:

> I talk about it, and I talk about it right away. Instead of having the kids wonder what the hell is going on, I

just tell them right out—explain why my face droops, why I limp, why there are certain sounds I have trouble producing. It works out well, and it usually leads to questions and answers. From that first-day activity it's amazing how the kids open up afterward. It's also amazing to me that more people don't share those kinds of experiences with each other. The kids look at me in awe and have a whole new attitude and respect that wasn't there before. They haven't been allowed that opportunity in the past.

Most people find that simple honesty—"matter-of-fact-ness"—is the best policy when dealing with the public. But first they have to come to grips with their illness, a process that can take years.

The Gift of Love and Support

You can't underestimate the part that your love and support play in your spouse's acceptance of the illness, ability to heal, quality of life, and even length of life. Frank, who has fought a long and courageous battle with lymphoma, is well aware of this:

> I could not have gotten through this by myself. If I'd been a single guy, with no strong caring and loving around, I never would have made it through this thing. I would have given up. I would have said, "This is not worth it. I don't have anything to look forward to even if I do get through this."

Sometimes that love and support must be delivered as a swift kick in the pants. After Sonya's husband became paralyzed she knew that jolting, not prodding, would have the greatest effect:

> At the beginning we were told there was a possibility that Jerry would be able to walk again, but it would depend primarily on his will. When we learned that

monumental fact I said to him, "If you do not try to recuperate, to be the very best that you can be through rehabilitation, but decide to rest on your laurels for the rest of your life, then I am leaving you *now*, because I would grow to hate you. I love you too much to let you do that to you and to me."

It took four long years, but the courage and strength Jerry displayed—with Sonya's prodding—cemented a marriage that might otherwise have foundered under the strain of a serious disability.

There is a song called "For Once in My Life (I Have Someone Who Needs Me)" that Michael sang to me for many years. When he got sick, I sang it to him. It reassured him that the "need" part of love and support was just as important to me as it had been to him. It was OK for him to be the one *in* need.

BEAR IN MIND:

Try to contain conversations about the illness. The illness can become so consuming that the caregiver soon grows weary of hearing about it.

Acknowledge that the patient's fear is real. Fear makes the ill person timid, reticent, tentative—or else a sudden daredevil.

Remember, it's not you the patient is angry with; it's the situation.

Help to alleviate the patient's guilt with constant reassurance. The crushing guilt can cause a patient to sacrifice too much.

Help the patient maintain contact with friends and family. Loss of a positive self-image can make a patient reclusive.

Be truthful. Most people find that simple honesty is the best policy when dealing with the public.

4
The Children

You are a mature, responsible adult, and yet at times you can't seem to cope with what has been happening at home since your partner in life became chronically ill. What about those members of your family who are even less well equipped to deal with a major change? What about the children?

Dr. Nancy Coniaris, a clinical psychologist, says, "I can't overestimate the amount of strain involved with a major chronic illness that goes on over a long period of time. It's very, very difficult on the adults who have to cope, and for the children it comes during the major, formative years of their lives. It gets woven into their very being."

For each child you have, the burden on you increases exponentially. Each age group brings its own set of problems. If you have tiny tots, your greatest difficulty might be in finding someone to help out or in dealing with their separation from you when a significant portion of your time must be devoted to someone else. If you have preteens, you might painfully watch them wrestle with fears they are unable to verbalize. Teenagers pose added complications; struggling through adolescence is hard enough without the strain of a sick parent adding to an already overburdened emotional load. And, as I discovered, even having grown children brings its own set of disappointments. My hope is that my vision is clearer as I look back so that I can offer some understanding and advice.

Unfulfilled Expectations

Between the two of us, Michael and I had six children. All of them were adults when he became ill, but that did not mean that everything went smoothly. Naturally, my greatest disappointment was that they didn't help out as much as I wished or hoped they would. They didn't fulfill my expectations.

Big kids aren't treated with kid gloves like little kids; ours were fully capable of realizing that Michael was going through a difficult time, but only when Michael was in the hospital did he seem to them to be clearly sick. At those times they visited him much more often than when he was at home. Coming by to see their father was difficult because—let's admit it—it was no fun visiting a sick, cranky parent. It was often difficult for them even to call, because all the old, unresolved family conflicts continued to get in the way. I thought that Michael's illness would put these into perspective and make them magically disappear but, if anything, it accentuated them.

I now realize that my expectations of volunteer help were unrealistic. Just as Michael had an insatiable need for me to be at home with him, so I had an insatiable need for our children to devote time to Michael. It was like a sieve, with water flowing out as fast as it was poured in. When an illness spans several years, you must work out a balance and learn to express how you feel. A friend of mine points out:

> As our parents grow into their seventies and eighties we begin to understand that we are expected to reverse roles and to care for them. In the new "sandwich generation," what children have the most difficulty with is watching a parent deteriorate in strength and health while still young. They often play ostrich and pretend it isn't happening: "If I don't go see Mom

and Dad, I won't notice how sick and weak they look this month."

What can you do if your children don't volunteer? Use them, to your advantage, whenever it is appropriate. For instance, when Michael went to Minnesota to be evaluated at the Mayo Clinic, I knew that the week would be filled with tests and appointments and that it was going to be a tough time because of the pending decision about the loss of his leg. I strongly encouraged one son, who lived out of town, to go along, and I stayed home. I wanted someone else to take over the responsibility for a little while.

Whenever Michael was in the hospital, I found myself staying away. That meant letting one day, perhaps even two, go by without a visit. I dealt with it alone at home all the time, and I figured that when he was in the hospital the other family members could pick up the slack.

Hiring your children is another way of getting their assistance and a much better way than nagging and harassing. Michael and I did this with three of ours. When one of the girls, who lived nearby, couldn't work for a time because of some dental work she was having done, we hired her to come over and cook dinner each evening. It was a terrific relief. On another occasion we lured the other daughter away from her job in another state to return for her final year of graduate school, which she was financing herself. We told her that we would pay for her schooling if she would live at home and be of help. She stayed for over a year. And one of the boys, who was the only one without a "go to work" type job, on several occasions came to work out of our home. We paid him for what he did to help us, because if he hadn't been available we would have had to pay someone else. Each situation was a blessing.

This same hiring tactic can be used with younger children. It is no different from saying, "I need gardening help this weekend. I need six hours of your time, but I won't make you do it for nothing. I'm going to pay you for it."

You can cut a middle ground that helps get things done but that doesn't take advantage of the child.

But I Just Had a Baby!

My children were grown, and yet they still complicated my situation with Michael. What happens if your children are small? How do you cope then?

Vanessa was eight months pregnant when her husband had an aneurysm that left him permanently brain-damaged:

> At the beginning I had two people at home, neither one of whom could turn over in bed, and I didn't know whose diapers to change first. I was totally exhausted.

Astute enough to realize that she couldn't cope on her own, Vanessa temporarily hired a nurse to help with the baby and then got herself a housekeeper. She also mobilized her family and friends. Since then Vanessa's life has not been easy, as you can well imagine. On the other hand, having the baby delivered along with the illness had its advantages:

> The baby was a comforting source of health and well-being, a sign that life goes on. And it gave Dennis a real focus in his therapy. One of the things they taught him in physical therapy was to pick the baby up. They would put a doll on the floor, have him kneel down and change its diaper, and then pick up the doll. The first time he was able to pick up the baby, it was a real accomplishment for him. The baby gave him something to live for, something to strive for.

Vanessa made an effort to let Dennis do everything he could do for the child without being critical about how it was done:

When helping a baby to eat, some people might get obsessed about how much is spilled on the floor. Dennis's motor coordination was not so great, nor was the baby's, but they had a great time, and I think we got enough spinach in her mouth to do some good. And if the bottle wasn't warmed properly or the diaper didn't get put on straight, what did it matter?

You have to relax your standards. In any marriage you have to learn to be able to accept the way the other person does things. When that person is a disabled spouse, you have to be consciously and constantly aware of letting that person do things to the best of his ability. You have to decide what's most important. To me, that meant allowing my daughter and her father to develop as normal a relationship as possible.

The Case for Honesty

Once past infancy, children serve as barometers of the emotional patterns around them. It might be tempting to protect yours by keeping the truth from them, but even very young children immediately sense any changes and tensions within the family. They are going to know by your behavior and even by your facial expressions if something is terribly wrong, and lies will only alienate them. Children will usually suffer far more from fear caused by what their imaginations might conjure up than they will from the truth.

They can be spared some of the messier details of an illness, especially if they are small, but if they are protected too much, serious repercussions may occur. When Louise was in the hospital for treatment of a brain tumor, her mother-in-law looked after the children:

> She told the kids they could not come up to the hospital and see me. I don't know why. Maybe she thought that they couldn't take it. I would have loved

to have seen them! And she told the kids not to cry in front of their father. I think that was a terrible thing to do!

In this family no one stood up to the well-meaning grandmother; consequently nothing was aired, nothing was shared. Now Louise is having drug and alcohol problems with her teenage daughter, and she is certain that the girl's behavior problems are a result of the family's inability to communicate during their time of terrible stress.

But sheltering our children from pain comes naturally to most of us. Even a reaction as extreme as a desire to escape, taking the children along, is not all that uncommon. Miranda and Arthur separated for a time after his illness became critical. There were many reasons for this, but one of them was a desire on her part to protect their baby:

> This may sound crazy, but I wanted to protect the child so that he didn't suffer a huge loss when his father died. Eventually I came to my senses. Even during the separation, Arthur and my son were seeing each other constantly, and both enjoyed each other thoroughly. Why would I rob this child of one moment with his father? I asked myself. We don't live in a perfect world. Let's be a family for as long as we can be, because a lot can be gained for all of us. When things get very difficult, when Arthur does get very ill and dies, then I'll handle that when the time comes.

Amy handled things at her house with total openness right from the first day her lupus was diagnosed:

> I've made a point of being straight with the kids, of including them. Initially, particularly when I was really, really sick, it was very scary. I didn't know what the next day was going to bring, what I'd be able to do or not do. I shared with them my fears, my concerns about what my lupus would mean.

I don't hide anything from them, although I don't always tell them all the gory details. And it's kind of age-appropriate. I don't say the same things to my seven-year-old as I do to my eleven-year-old and my thirteen-year-old. For my seven-year-old, it's more a question of dealing with the idea that if you have a parent who gets sick, could they die, and what's going to happen? It's been hardest on her in that she's at that in-between age where she's beginning to understand what an illness is about, but doesn't really. She felt pretty threatened by the whole thing, had a lot of anxiety about what was going to happen to me. I coped with her anxiety by just talking to her a lot, very openly.

Joyce was also open with her children. Her husband underwent minor surgery during which a malignant tumor was unexpectedly discovered, and when she came home that night, still in a state of fear and shock, she didn't try to shelter anyone:

I told them the truth, that a tumor had been found and that things were much more serious than expected and that the doctors were doing tests. They were told each step of the way what was happening and what could happen. We talked about what he had and we used the proper terminology, from cancer to tumor. They knew everything. I didn't want them going to school and having someone say, "I hear your father has cancer" and not being aware of that.

The oldest, who was in seventh grade, was aware that cancer frequently meant death. She felt the most afraid, although she didn't really express it. I'm sure they were scared just seeing him, because it *was* scary. *I* was scared seeing him that way. The younger ones probably didn't have a concept of what might or might not happen. I think they were reassured that this illness and the radiation were temporary and that their dad would get better when the radiation stopped, and so there was a time period in there which they could understand.

Jesse's wife developed a dangerous heart condition and had a stroke when their children were aged four, seven, nine, and thirteen:

> I never held back anything about it. I never lied to them at any time. There were no secrets. Because she was a stroke victim, they could see that she was different than before, so I had to tell them why. I didn't scare them; I just tried to tell them in such a way that they would understand, presenting it to them in their own language.
>
> I told them she was going to get better because we were all going to help her. We would help Mommy with her physical therapy and with her speech, help her breathe and make her work on saying words. They all felt they contributed to making it better.
>
> They had very little fear. And they knew exactly what to do each time she had a heart attack and how to do it without going into a panic. If I was at work or out of town, one would get on the phone and immediately call the ambulance, and the others would get her into a comfortable position. It wasn't because they were taught: it was education by association, all the being around and listening and having dialogue about it.

Warning Signals

Because Jesse kept the lines of communication open, his children faced their mother's fragile condition in a healthy manner. But for many children the worry of having an ill parent manifests itself in some behavioral manner. Depression is one, and depression is not inappropriate. You are probably depressed, too. If your child seems sad, listless, lost in his or her own little world, or full of aches and pains, these are all common reactions to the changing situation at home.

But sadness can also be acted out in other ways that are more difficult to decipher. *Depressive equivalence* is the term given to sadness that is replaced or masked by other behaviors that at first don't seem to be directly related to the stress at home. It can occur at any age. Michael's and my children went through periods of nonmotivation at work and at first had trouble figuring out why. Once they understood the problem, they constructed their own support networks among friends and coworkers, and I was amazed to see just how extensive these networks became.

Depressive equivalence is often seen in children. The following behaviors might be warning signals that something is wrong:

- Changes in appetite
- Dropping grades in school
- Wildness and irresponsibility
- Fears and phobias, often relating to school
- Changes in behavior that are negative and nonproductive
- Difficulty functioning with people
- Eating and sleeping problems
- Low self-esteem

Rather than showing depression, a teenager might start raising hell. Drinking, driving around too fast, and getting involved prematurely in sex can all be ways of pushing away from the emotional discomfort at home. Dr. Coniaris explains why:

> The emotional pain involved in the whole situation is so unbearable that the kids will do almost anything they can to medicate themselves out of the mood that they're in, whether with drinking or getting involved prematurely in sex or smoking a lot of grass. Any kind of behavioral disturbance in kids—truancy or declining grades or increased drug or alcohol use or irresponsible behavior with cars—is a way the kid is trying to cope with the stress, anxiety, pain, and parental preoccupation with the illness.

The stresses on a child whose parent is sick or dying can

make drugs even more tempting than they might otherwise be. And if a child—teenaged or grown—turns to drugs during the time that a parent is chronically ill, the issue is even touchier than usual because the patient might feel responsible. That happened in our family, and Michael felt angry and totally responsible. In a way he was, because his illness was a factor contributing to the stress in our children's lives. He had a hard time dealing with that issue.

What Can You Do?

What can you do if your children show signs of serious stress? The first step is to *keep an open pipeline*. Find out what is going on in their lives and encourage them to be open by being open about your own feelings. One of the things that you have to watch out for is that you don't focus all your attention on the sick person at the expense of the children. It is vital to allocate a certain amount of time to helping the kids deal with all the emotional implications that arise when one parent is sick or disabled.

But when there is a serious illness that goes on for a long period of time, you are so overloaded with coping, sometimes just with the day-to-day medical care of your spouse, that dealing with the emotional part of it is way beyond what you have the strength to do. The kids very easily get the message that they shouldn't discuss it, so they don't deal with their own emotions in a direct way. They don't discuss it with anybody, assuming that if the family can't talk about it, then nobody should.

It is important to be aware that if emotions and problems aren't dealt with, they won't go away; they will simply come out in another form at another time. If you are already overloaded and don't seem to have time for your children, make sure that someone else is available—a favorite uncle, perhaps, or a grandparent.

Educate the family about the illness and its accompanying emotional strain. There are many books available, even for small children, that deal with feelings and with illness, even with death. Don't underestimate your child's capacity to understand. "My thirteen-year-old has actually read some of the books I have about my disease," says one mother, "and has a pretty good understanding about what's going on."

Involve your children in the caretaking to help them feel a part of a solid family structure. During the eight weeks of isolation that accompanied her father's bone-marrow transplant, Stacy saw neither parent because at the time they thought it would be too much for her to deal with. "It was even frightening for me to look at all the stuff I was hooked up to," says her father. "And I lost forty-plus pounds; I was a bag of bones. I really looked like I'd been through whatever I'd been through."

In retrospect, Stacy's mother has changed her mind about her protective attitude:

> The mistake that I made was in not insisting that Stacy be more a part of it. If I were advising someone who had a teenage child—and it would have to be someone that old to understand the setting, the germfree environment, and all—I would insist that they come and spend at least one night a week down there, being the caretaker, and be in the room a lot more.

Change family activities if one parent is restricted in physical activity. Otherwise there will be a lot of Because Ofs,—a lot of saying, "We can't go to the lake because Dad can't go with us" or "We can't take a vacation because of Mom's illness." *The caregiver has to be very careful that the children don't come to resent the Foreverness to the point where they begin to hope it will end.*

The family can have fun even though one parent is bedridden, and he or she can still be a part of it all. There are many things that can be done with the entire family or with individual children. Reading aloud, playing games, or just talking and cuddling will help to maintain a close-knit family structure. Jesse's family is a good example:

> The only thing my children were deprived of was their mother's activity. She couldn't play ball or go swimming or run around in the street with them, but she was always with them, she always participated simply by being there. What developed from that was a closer relationship between her and the kids.

Children—even big ones—don't always know what to say around a sick parent, so help your children find activities or topics of conversation to share. Some safe harbors are activities that the kids are involved in, crossword puzzles, books currently being read, or politics (although in some families this one might not be too safe!). One of my sons is a sports nut, so he always talked about sports with Michael. It was a good, continuing subject.

Create mini-events to give the kids something to do with or around the patient. Have a picnic. Pack up a lunch and have a party in the patient's hospital room or bedroom. Decorate with balloons if there's not already a birthday, holiday, or other occasion to set the theme.

Maximize your support system. Sometimes the only thing that saves children from permanent damage is that, when they lose one parent, the rest of the system is still working. Because the surviving parent will be absorbed with grief, he or she may not have enough energy to help the children through their grief, too, so it becomes vitally important that other friends and relatives step in to fill the gap. The same is true during illness if the parents are short of time to spend with the kids. It's critical that you make the most of your family and friends, trying to maximize everyone's impact on the children through visits, doing things together, and being together on holidays.

Use your support system for yourself, too, as Vanessa did:

> I never had any hesitancy about letting the baby go to

my mother's, an hour away, to spend the night. My health was paramount, too. I was recovering not only from childbirth but also from six weeks of exhaustion from Dennis's being in intensive care. I let the baby go to my mother's for the weekend when she was two months old, and since then she has continued to go one weekend a month.

Inform the school so that teachers will be sympathetic and realize that the children are going to be in a fragile emotional state. If the reason for behavioral problems or failing grades is understood in advance, these can be dealt with before they get out of hand.

In elementary school the teacher can be informed directly, but the best approach is often through the guidance counselor. Even elementary schools often have a trained professional on staff. The role of the guidance counselor becomes even more important in junior high and high school, when students have not one but many teachers.

Get professional help if necessary. If your children's problems are serious and persistent and seem beyond your ability to cope, it's time to consider some outside assistance. How to go about finding the best possible help is discussed in Chapter 15.

Keep the family laughing. When Michael was in the hospital and lost interest in taking care of himself, the kids would shave him. They'd prop him up in the bed and go at him with his electric razor, ribbing him like mad. You could see that even through all his desperation he was smiling inside, and it wouldn't have mattered if they were five years old or fifty—they were just kids playing with Daddy.

Humor is a valuable tool for lightening the atmosphere at home. Laughter is a natural outlet, providing a release from tension. Jesse says that his children find that teasing their mother helps to stifle their fears:

> My wife sometimes has a tough time in forming words, so we play "Twenty Questions" with her. Or when she stutters, we say, "Go ahead, say what you

want to say, let it all out," as if she's purposely holding back.

She joins right in on the fun. And if one of the kids is acting up, she'll taunt, "Don't aggravate me, or the next one might be my Big One." She is not in any way hesitant to use her condition, to joke about it or to use it to make a point about something. She will say to the kids, "I didn't raise you so that I could die of a heart attack worrying about you. If I am going to have a heart attack, let it be for my own reasons, not yours."

Whatever the age of your children, *periodically take the emotional temperature* of each one. Make a date to go out together, just the two of you. Whether you go to a nice restaurant or to Burger King, your "date" will give you a chance to do three things: to enjoy each other without guilt, to see how each other is doing, and to spend time alone together.

Hidden Fears

Fear can run rampant in families dealing with chronic illness. You probably have a whole list of fears yourself, from fear of losing your best friend, companion, and lover to fear that your personal being will be swallowed up by the unending burden of caregiving. One man I spoke with even admitted to fears that his son will think less of him—actually lose respect for him—because he is sick and might die.

You know what your own fears are because you are an adult and hopefully in tune with yourself, but with children many fears remain hidden. Perhaps the worst is that *the sick parent will die,* and there's frequently enough to it that you can't just soothe those fears away.

Stacy was in the eighth grade when her father was diagnosed as having lymphoma. Her mother describes the stress that it caused:

It was very scary for her. She went through a time where she really didn't want to face it. The first two or three years, when she was just hit with it—*pow,* this is what it can be like, this is what it looks like when you really go down—she would choose not to think about it for a while or not to put herself in a position where she might cry in front of a friend or in front of a classmate. She would avoid that at all costs.

By the time Stacy was fifteen her father had already undergone radiation and chemotherapy without success. The last resort was a bone marrow transplant:

That's when things got really, really horrible for her. She knew there was a chance that he could die. The day I told Stacy that her daddy had decided to go through the bone-marrow transplant, she cried and said, "But I wanted him to be alive for my high-school graduation."

And my response to her was, "We're doing this so that he can. But Stacy, I can't offer you any guarantees, and I promise you that even if he's not alive, you will graduate. And everybody who loves you will be there. You will go on." Difficult as it may be, you must constantly affirm that life will continue, that your children's goals and happiness will not come to an end with the death of a parent.

Connected to the fear of the sick parent dying is the fear that *the caregiver parent will die, too.* A child who has experienced the death of one parent or the fear that accompanies the illness of a parent can't take it for granted that the other parent will be OK. He needs constant reassurance.

A third hidden fear experienced by children is the *contagion factor*: Will I get the same condition? If the disease is a hereditary one, such as Alzheimer's or diabetes, this fear is very real. Part of the reason that Michael's two daughters are so concerned about exercise and diet may be because of a hidden fear of getting diabetes.

But the fear of contagion can be strong even if the illness

has no genetic implications or if the chronic condition was caused by an accident rather than an illness. With children this fear can take on an almost superstitious quality, particularly if other tragedies have taken place during the same time span as the parent's illness: "If Mommy is sick, Grandpa died, and my brother broke his arm, then Daddy and I must be next in line for something bad to happen." Once again, the child needs constant reassurance and help in seeing his lack of logic.

The fear of contagion, when based upon genetic reality, can take the form of a dangerous form of denial. Michael's two sons, who closely resemble him in physical characteristics and life-style, are or have been smokers, are overweight, and are not diet conscious. They deny that what happened to their father could happen to them too, and their denial is so massive that it might succeed in bringing their most hidden fear to a grim reality.

Another type of hidden fear is that *the child caused the illness*. This fear usually shows up as guilt. A child who has acted up may feel responsible for a parent's illness, particularly if it is something on the order of a heart condition:

> We had a son who had a drug problem, and he felt the guiltiest. "Do you think what I did made Dad sick?" the boy would ask. My husband didn't realize that's what his son was feeling, or if he did, he didn't go that extra little bit to make him feel better.

Fear in grown children can manifest itself as a refusal to face and accept the illness of a parent. This most often occurs when the parent has a cognitive disability. Frances struggled for eight years with a husband whose Alzheimer's disease caused his mental functions to deteriorate rapidly. She desperately needed help from her son, but he had none to give:

> My son Jason couldn't accept the fact that there was something wrong with his father. Whenever I tried to

unburden myself to him and his wife, tried to get them to realize the traumatic time I was having, they would say, "If you're going to be complaining the way you are, we're not coming home anymore." Jason never understood until the day his father did not know who he was. That almost killed Jason. He cried like a baby for two hours because he finally realized that his father was very ill.

Counseling and support groups are vital in a situation like Frances's. Just the knowledge that someone believes what she is saying and understands what she is going through can be of tremendous relief and will help her to feel that she is not alone.

What's the best way of coping with the other hidden fears? "Talking about it," says Dr. Coniaris. "Open pipelines make it less likely that the kid is going to shove the anxiety under, where it will fester until it starts coming out in another form." If the prognosis is bad, it's best to let them know that something drastic may happen but that you're still hoping and praying and getting treatment. Most importantly of all, search out those hidden fears, talk openly about them, and give as much reassurance as you can.

Money Matters

Another hidden fear that can occur when a parent's illness is terminal, and that can surface either before or after the parent dies, concerns inheritance. Money, particularly inherited money, is a concern that begins unconsciously creeping into everybody's mind whenever a parent is sick or dying. Left to its own devices, it can become an evil and insidious matter that can permeate all relationships within the family.

If one grown child takes on more than his or her share of helping with the caretaking—whether for reasons of close proximity, better abilities, or a greater sense of responsibility—it is natural for the other children to start to worry about their inheritance. The chief worry is usually that the care-giving child will wind his way into the heart of the sick parent to the extent of affecting the will. Meanwhile, the care-giving child resents the siblings who don't help, and so the stage is set for some serious family strife.

This situation becomes even more potentially explosive when both natural and stepchildren are involved, particularly if a stepchild is still at home when the natural children are not. And if a natural parent is ill but the stepparent is quite well, the children can't help but wonder what will happen to them when their natural parent dies. There can be a great deal of hidden fear relating to a stepparent who might get married again and to an inheritance that might slip away.

You must thoroughly investigate all background scenarios and figure out what might backfire. You need to recognize that what the children are feeling is a fear of losing what they think should be theirs. Watch out for the calm before the storm, or you may discover too late, as I did, that there are some hidden fears and jealousies developing without your children even knowing it.

Clearly address this subject well ahead of time. *Sit down with your children—and your sick spouse if possible—and discuss the issue of money.* Help the children understand what has been set up, and why. They needn't be told all the details of the will, but they should know generally what to expect so there won't be any surprises and so they don't begin to develop any unrealistic ideas of what is coming to them. *Sit down with them one-on-one*, not as a group, so that any fears can be easily expressed.

"Bad" Emotions

Many people are shocked by the feelings they have. Teens, in particular, must deal with an unfamiliar and scary range of emotions. They may be angry at the sick parent for what he or she has done to the family life or be resentful that the care-giving parent no longer has much attention to give them. The "bad" feelings are then followed by crushing guilt.

"I'm so selfish," a high-school boy might think. "My dad is dying of cancer, and all I can think about is whether I'll be able to go to that party Saturday night." He is shocked that his daily needs take precedence over the seriousness of the problem at home. He thinks he should be sad and serious, but his mind refuses to focus on the subject at hand and instead drifts off to the upcoming party. Psychiatrist John Coniaris explains:

> If a child thinks he should be sad or grieving, but his mind won't stick to the appropriate subject, it is easy for him to become worried about his state of mental health if he is not aware that this type of mental activity is perfectly normal. Even many adults are not aware of the degree that the mind bounces around and do not realize that even in the midst of a tragic situation the mind will be at ease from time to time, going right back to the daily routines of normal existence. A teenager, whose self-esteem is often low anyway, can quickly lose what's left of it if he's embarrassed about the thoughts running through his head.

Anger is another emotion that can affect a child greatly, even though anger is an appropriate response to an unfair blow struck by life. When Stacy's father was fighting his cancer, she was consumed by anger—a great deal of anger that was expressed, according to her mother, in typical teenage ways of rebelling:

> It was primarily in attitude and lack of cooperativeness. There weren't any drugs or staying out all night or any of the major things that you worry about. It was all attitudinal.
> Stacy had a hard time, a real hard time. It affected her emotionally. She carried things off physically; she looked OK on the outside, and to a casual acquain-

tance or to friends and family members she appeared to be pretty much together. But after we all got back home from the hospital, I began to realize that she was in pretty bad shape.

With a long-term illness children can actually reach a point where they begin to resent the sick parent for getting all the attention and for making home life miserable. They might eventually start hoping that the parent will die and get it over with, and that type of thinking is then followed by terrible guilt. Dr. Nancy Coniaris suggests how to deal with this:

> It's the same problem that a lot of adults have. There's a lot of thinking like that—it's inevitable. It's better if you're relatively conscious that that's what you're thinking and that it's understandable under the circumstances, that you're not a monster for wishing that your parent would just die.

Stacy, says her mother, was fortunately able to express herself:

> Once, when things were going badly, Stacy said to me, "Mama, it seems so hard. Do you ever think sometimes that it would be easier if Daddy just died?" I said, "Yes, Stacy, sometimes I think that. But in my heart I know that is not true, that his being here with us is important, that the essence of him is important to us. It might be easier not to have to go through some of this, but it's never better when somebody dies, because that person, if you have a close relationship, is so important to you and to your wholeness that to be without him leaves a void." She could understand that.

Even adults will succumb to "bad" emotions. Many of those parents who dealt with their family crises in a healthy manner expressed a certain amount of guilt over

some of their own emotional reactions to stress. "I sometimes take out my frustrations on my son," says one
mother. "When he does something wrong I bring it up that
his dad's so sick, and then I hate myself afterwards."

Another mother admits to similar problems:

> I can remember once getting mad at my daughter.
> She was getting sort of flippant, and she said some-
> thing pretty bad about her father. I told her that her
> dad was really sick, so sick that he might die, and she
> had better remember that. I struck out at her because
> she was the easiest target when she was at me and I
> was at her. I felt awful afterward, because she already
> knew it and she didn't need to be told in that way. I
> felt more guilty, I think, over that argument than
> over anything else. I told her later that I felt bad, and
> we talked about it.

The sick parent is angry, too, and often directs much of
that anger toward the family. It is easy for a parent to get
frustrated even in a normal parent-child relationship, but
the ill parent is going to lash out more because he's feeling
more helpless and has fewer reserves. You are adult
enough to understand this, but your children may need
some help in identifying the source of that frightening
wrath.

Responsibility Promotes Growth

The potential problems looming in your future may at
times seem overwhelming, but that doesn't mean that only
gloom and doom lie ahead. Jesse stresses some of the
positive effects that came about when his children were
given new responsibilities:

> We all pitched in and did everything ourselves. The
> kids were very responsible. The oldest boy took
> charge and the other children would help him. We
> used to make dinners and freeze them so that each
> evening the kids could just take something out of the

freezer and throw it in the oven. When I came home from work they would have the table set and all the goodies popped in the middle of it.

Whatever we had to do, we just got it done. They knew that their mother was in a position that she needed help, and they proceeded to be responsible. Unto this day I never had a problem with my kids in that area. They all realized they had a certain amount of responsibility, and they lived up to it.

It helps smooth things out when everybody knows they can do a little bit to help the situation. They had to be more alert, to watch their mother and look for signs of trouble. She would never tell me if she was feeling bad. When I came home the kids would say, "Hey, Dad, you had better check with Mom because she hasn't been herself. She has been moping around—maybe there is something wrong with her." A condition like my wife's puts a little bit more responsibility on the children than normal, but it was for the better.

Amy agrees about the benefits of added responsibilities:

I've been pleased with how the kids have been able to help out and understand and be supportive. During the worst of my illness, the oldest two were capable of getting things together, getting meals, doing things that needed to be done. We have a grocery store that's close by that they could walk to and that sort of thing. In some ways it's been a good experience for them to have to rely more on themselves, to be able to use the strengths they have in order to deal with the situation.

Even young children can be educated to share some of the responsibilities and concerns of a parent's illness. Arthur's lung disease requires him to breathe oxygen nearly twenty-four hours a day:

My two-and-a-half-year-old probably thinks that all daddies have oxygen. That's been part of me as long

as he's known me, and I don't think it's registered yet
that there's anything unusual in that regard. He
knows that I'm sick, and he brings my medicine to me
in the morning before I get up.

My eight-year-old understands much better what
my illness means, and he can be sensitive in some
ways pretty far beyond his years. A couple of years
ago, when he was six, we went to a park with a
vertical elevation of 100 or 150 feet from the parking
lot to the top. It's a gradual slope, but for me that's a
challenge. He and I walked up, and by the time we got
to the top I was really out of breath. He said, "Let's sit
here awhile." It wasn't as though I needed to sit
down, it was as though he needed to sit down, and
why didn't I sit down with him? He told me later that
he knew I wanted to breathe and rest. At six years
old!

It is not easy to be a good parent and a good caregiver all
at the same time, but in spite of your already laden plate of
responsibilities, it is up to you to bring the family to peace.
There are three steps necessary to accomplish this. The first is to
talk, to maintain that open pipeline. The second is to keep
your eyes open to warning signals that mean your child
needs help. The third is to get that help, whether it comes
from you, from a friend or relative, or from a professional.

As with most interpersonal relationships, communication is the key to success. Be open, be honest, be persistent,
and offer help. Try to see things through the eyes of your
children.

If your children are grown and the help is resisted, put it
on the list of things you cannot control and stop worrying
about it. But if you do succeed, the rewards can be great.
During Michael's illness, one of his daughters invited me—
just me, alone—to a nice restaurant for dinner. The occasion was that she wanted an opportunity to tell me this: "I
know what you are going through. I know what you are
doing, and I also know that if you weren't doing it, I would
have to be doing it. I want you to know how much I love

you and appreciate you, and I also want you to know that I am going to try to do better."

What more can a parent ask for?

BEAR IN MIND:

Pay your children to help care for the patient. Hiring your children is better than nagging and harassing.

Do not lie to your children about the illness. Children serve as barometers of the emotional patterns around them and will sense any changes or tension.

Be careful that the children don't come to resent the Foreverness to the point where they begin to hope it will end.

Periodically take the emotional temperature of each child.

Maintain open communication to help dispel the fear that can run rampant in families dealing with chronic illness.

Don't be afraid to ask for help. Even young children can be educated to share some of the responsibilities and concerns of a parent's illness.

5
Friends and Relatives: Your First Line of Support

I never expected that being a caregiver would teach me lessons in being a friend. I didn't realize what was happening until about a year after the doctors had removed Michael's first leg. When I looked back, I became aware that I had begun to relate to people in a new and different way.

As an entrepreneur, I was always the motivator in any business I was connected with. One of the motivator's main functions is to maintain a positive outlook and assure other people associated with a given project that it's going to succeed with flying colors. Like most businesspeople, I had been a very private person in matters relating to my personal life. Because of the stress I was under, however, I began sharing events in my personal life with friends and business associates I felt close to. I would say, for instance, "Michael's back in the hospital again." And the other person would say something like, "Oh, I'm so sorry" or "Would you like to tell me about it?" or "How are *you* holding up through all this?" I soon learned that I could tell by a person's response whether he or she was really interested and wanted to know more.

When I became aware of what I was doing, I was really surprised. I remember thinking, "That's not at all like me." I had been used to talking about business or about people, places, and things, but it was rare to get to the feeling level in any conversation. Now, suddenly, I was aware that I was disclosing feelings, putting myself at peril in a sense, and seeing who tossed out a life raft. A lot of people did. And many of them shared their own feelings with me in return.

I even began to share personal events in speeches, using them as background material that added weight to the main theme. I remember the first time I did it, shortly after Michael lost his first leg. The speech was about overcoming roadblocks to power. The particular roadblock I was discussing was the danger of letting outside circumstances consume all your energies and attention. When I mentioned the recent compounding of personal events, including Michael's loss of his leg, I could hear a sound in the audience like one collective indrawn breath. I got a standing ovation at the end of the speech. A number of people came up and spoke to me afterward, as was usually the case after I had given a talk, but this time many mentioned personal tragedies of their own—a divorce, the loss of a child, whatever. I found from such experiences that I could draw reinforcement and strength from sharing.

Your Best Support Group Is Closer Than You Think

It's an accepted fact that maintaining a network of friends can make a vital contribution to a chronically ill person's quality of life. Dr. Kitty Stein, a psychologist who counsels a number of multiple-sclerosis patients, says:

> At one point I actually stopped seeing a woman in treatment because I felt like therapy wasn't what she wanted. What she wanted was friends. The chronically ill person needs friends. The caregiver also needs a support system, sometimes very separate from the patient's.

A striking number of caregivers we interviewed listed friends and/or relatives as their main network of support.

Joyce's husband fought a cancer battle that put an enormous amount of strain on her, too:

> My friends and family made more of a difference in my ability to cope with this than anything else I can think of. It was wonderful having people I could turn to, real people who weren't embroiled in what was happening with the situation like I was. I could talk about it when I needed to. There were a lot of times I felt like withdrawing, but if I had just lived with my thoughts and my sick spouse, that would have been awful.

Of priceless value is the friend who, after inquiring about the condition of your chronically ill husband or wife, then asks quietly, "And now how are *you*?" Such friends and relatives form your important link with the real world out there that keeps on turning, the world apart from your isolation and your spouse's suffering. They give you a listening ear and a shoulder to cry on. They also provide the positive strokes a caregiver needs, all the way from "That color looks good on you" to "You're an inspiration to us all."

Particularly close friends or relatives can serve an important function as monitors, keeping in touch with you regularly to make sure you really *are* doing OK. It is an enormous comfort to know they are there. Really close friends can sometimes monitor both you and your spouse—as well as your marriage—with deep sensitivity. Katy, who has had severe asthma all her life, knows the value of friends:

> I have a close friend who knows us well enough as a married couple that she can stabilize us at the crisis point. Whichever of us is having the problem, she can get us through it and be supportive. To get a third party like that is not always easy, but it's extremely helpful.

Having close friends or family members who understand your situation and your spouse's condition can often make possible a social life for the two of you that would be difficult or impossible under other circumstances. Ben, a corporate executive whose wife has lupus, is an example:

> Our social life has been impacted, there's no denying that, but our supportive circle of friends has made things a lot easier. They're always very understanding if we have to leave early or if we have to make special accommodations for Cynthia. If we are out at someone's home, everyone is keeping an eye on her for any sign that she's about to fade, and they are equipped to offer her a place to lie down or whatever. We still stay socially busy and just work around any problems her illness creates.

Let Yourself Be Cared For

Face it. When you're a caregiver, you're really *not* fine all the time. I wasn't, and I doubt that anyone is. But if you don't let other people know that, they won't be able to help you. If there's one overriding thing I want to emphasize, it's that you have to let yourself be cared for. If you don't provide the opportunity, there's nothing anyone can do for you.

Many people feel helpless in the face of other people's adversity. That is particularly true if they have never had to cope with similarly devastating situations in their own lives. Your closest friends may be deeply affected by what has happened to you and your spouse and may be overwhelmingly sorry. They may want desperately to help, but they don't know where to begin. They don't even know what questions to ask—or if it's appropriate to ask questions at all. In the face of such obstacles, these friends may simply disappear from your life, surfacing only for stilted telephone Courtesy Calls every month or so.

This doesn't have to happen. And there are steps you can

take to see that it doesn't. All you need to do is show these people how they can help you and let them know specifically what they can do.

It may be something as simple as telling them, during one of their Courtesy Calls, that you really like to hear from them. Be specific about what you enjoy talking about. For example, say, "It's really so good for me to hear about your children and your family. It gets me outside my own problems. I hope you'll call me again soon with more news."

In order to make friends or relatives feel comfortable with your situation, you may also have to guide them regarding what they can ask you about. For example, people could ask me anything about Michael's condition; I usually didn't mind talking about it at all. If for some reason I didn't want to answer something or perhaps was weary of explaining the same thing for the fortieth time, I'd let them know. One family tackled this problem by writing a detailed letter explaining the illness, the treatment, what they did and didn't want to talk about, and specific topics to be avoided in front of their small children. They mailed copies of the letter to all their friends and work associates. But even if I occasionally didn't want to talk about Michael's condition, I was always glad that someone had cared enough to ask, and I told them that.

"If there's anything I can do . . ." is an easy phrase to say, and in a crisis many people say it. For some people it's simply a matter of form. For others, however, it's a heartfelt offer. Ironically, it's usually an offer that goes unheeded, often in the face of great need. Good friends would truly like to help. They simply don't know how. And our problem as caregivers is that we don't know how—or are afraid—to ask them.

After Michael had had several setbacks and I had heard this phrase from a number of people, I sat down one day and made a list of ways these people *could* help. The next time I heard "If there's anything I can do . . ." I was able to answer immediately, "Oh yes, there *is*. You can come keep Michael company some evening while I go out by myself to

dinner and a movie," or any one of several other needs I
had identified that they could fill.

Vanessa did this even better than I:

> When people said, "What can I do?" I made them put
> their money where their mouth was. I said, "I'm in
> desperate need of a new housecoat. Would you go out
> and buy me one?" or "Dennis needs some pajamas,"
> or "Dennis needs some slip-on shoes." I was very
> specific. I found out very quickly who was sincere
> about offering help and who was just giving lip ser-
> vice. And once you help people, it makes them feel
> better because they are able to be of service.
>
> What I wound up appreciating most was the person
> who would come, look around, and say, "Hmmm, you
> look like you could do with a load of laundry. Why
> don't I do it for you?" My family was very good at
> that. My mother went out and bought me a new trash
> can one day because mine leaked. Somebody else
> went in and cleaned up my kitchen. I also asked
> people to come in and baby-sit or to take Dennis out.

Everybody's needs are different. You may, for instance,
be able to tell one friend she can grocery-shop for you the
next time she goes to the store or another friend that he
can provide needed transportation to a physical-therapy
session one day over lunch hour. Short, uncomplicated
favors and errands are best, and you should not ask more
than one at a time in order to make it clear that you do not
intend to impose on anyone.

One more thing you have to do in order to allow your
friends to care for you is make time for *them*. This is
particularly difficult for the working caregiver. The duties
of caregiving frequently demand at least as much time as a
part-time job, and that's time you put in over and above
your regular full-time employment.

I have found, though, that it is possible to carve out little
niches of time to spend with friends even when you work.
One friend and I took a walk during lunch or after work
instead of having a meal. That gave us a chance to be alone

and talk. I also began inviting friends to join me when I worked out at the end of the business day and then had a salad with them afterward. That gave us even more time. In neither case did this cut into the time I would have spent with Michael.

Different Kinds of Friends
Provide Different Kinds of Support

I found myself dividing people into categories based on how often I saw or talked to them and the depth of support they were able to give me. Then I thought about relatives outside my immediate family and discovered that the same thing held true: different relatives were fulfilling different functions in my life in relation to my situation with Michael.

I would like to pass on to you the categories of friends and relatives I arrived at. I imagine that if you do this exercise, yours will be much the same.

1. *The Very Best.* These were my closest confidantes. For me it was a category of two. Both lived in my hometown of Atlanta, which made them more available when I needed to talk. And we could talk about our feelings openly and honestly, without pretense on either side. These were not necessarily the people I had been friends with the longest, although we had been close for at least a year or two before Michael became ill. Our friendships deepened after that.

There is a poignant point for discussion here. In so many instances it is your spouse who has been your best friend. Michael and I were lucky because our friendship stood the test of his illness. Sometimes, however, chronic illness can alter such a friendship forever. An extreme case is Vanessa, whose husband suffered severe brain trauma after a cerebral aneurysm. His personality is now significantly altered:

> We were in the same field. Dennis had always been my mentor. He had extraordinary respect, as well as extraordinary experience, so I was accustomed to

asking his advice. Now all of a sudden he agrees with me about everything. He's emotionally dependent on other people to set the tone in a gathering. He has trouble sorting out his own feelings from whatever is going on around him, and he will parrot my opinion. That makes me feel really lonesome, really alone in the world. It's kind of like an unrequited love affair. I can't get over him, because—it's like that old song— "there's always something there to remind me." His face is still the same, but he's not there.

2. *Extremely Close but Living in Distant Cities.* Had these friends lived in Atlanta, they probably would have ranked among the very best. When we were together we were extremely open about what we were feeling, but we may have had such conversations only once a month or so, depending on how often I was in their cities or on the frequency of long-distance phone calls.

3. *Long-Term Friends.* These were people I had known for years and whom I would have regarded as my closest friends before Michael's illness. We remained close and I could express my feelings easily with them. Although we didn't talk very often, when we did we'd talk for hours. I knew they were there if I needed them.

4. *Genuinely Good Buddies.* These were mostly business friends and there were maybe two dozen of them, equal numbers of men and women. We would go to dinner, go to lunch at meetings, or have a cocktail after work. We would get together for business reasons and subsequently talk about personal matters. I don't think I appreciated at the time what a very important mainstay they were. They kept normality in my life. And because there were so many of them, such a big base, these were the people I turned to when I feared others of my friends might be growing tired of the responsibility of caring for a caregiver.

5. *Friends of Your Spouse.* I divided these into three sub-categories:

(a) *The Very Best.* These were people who were always there for Michael with a call or a visit and who knew how to show they cared.

(b) *Those Who Cared a Lot but Didn't Know How to Show It.*
They would send a card or letter that said as much: "I'm
sorry I haven't been by, but I really don't know what I can
do." Perhaps the best illustration in this category comes
from Katy:

> One of the nicest things that ever happened to me
> was when a girlfriend of mine didn't know how to
> deal with it when I was going through a bad time. She
> couldn't verbalize anything, but she just put a card—
> it didn't matter what it was, not necessarily a get-well
> card—in the mail. She only signed her name. It
> showed me that she might not be able to talk to me,
> but she was thinking of me in a demonstrative way. It
> was her way of showing that she cared. I'll never
> forget that for nearly two months I got something in
> the mail every single day. That takes some doing.

(c) *Michael's Friends Who Disappointed Me.* These were
people who had been extremely close to Michael but suddenly didn't call and didn't come around. They were very
conspicuous by their absence.

Your Spouse's Friend or Relative Who Disappoints

Almost everyone we interviewed mentioned, with either
sadness, resentment, or resignation, that there had been at
least one friend of the chronically ill spouse who had
disappointed them. Allen is a high-school teacher who had
a cerebellar tumor. Its surgical removal left him with a
speech impediment, visual problems, partial facial paraly-
sis, and coordination problems:

> When I was in the hospital, it was interesting who
> came to visit and who didn't. That was an eye-
> opener. Some people I was fairly close to did come in,
> but then there were others who did not. Not a lot did.
> It's possible they didn't know how to respond to what
> was going on with me. I can understand that to a
> certain extent. I know it's difficult for some people,

but I think friendship should have gotten them over that hurdle.

I remember my father coming in and having some real problems with that, too. Here I am lying on the bed with a 99 percent chance of dying shortly, and he's talking to me about the weather. I yelled, "For Christ's sake, Dad, I've gotta figure out what to do with my wife and son if I die!" He just kind of broke down and couldn't accept it, and left.

My greatest disappointment was Ray, the man who had been Michael's closest friend for the longest time. Ray and Michael had vacationed together every year for twenty years until Michael became too ill. When Michael lost his first leg, Ray just disappeared. I really couldn't handle that, and I couldn't figure out why it had happened. Ray had remarried the year before, and I thought perhaps his disappearance had to do with his wife, that maybe he didn't want to look back and bring sadness into this new life. But it really bothered me, and of course it bothered Michael.

One day when Michael was in the hospital, a good three years into his illness and after he had lost his other leg, Ray made one of his stilted and infrequent Courtesy Calls. He was then living in California. I told him, "Ray, I want you to know I'm really disappointed in you. I hope I don't hurt you, but I am hurt, and I want to tell you why." I went on to tell him everything I was feeling. By the time I was finished, I was sobbing over the phone and so was he. He acknowledged that he had been unable to deal with what had happened to Michael, and he was ashamed of himself for it. He was relieved that I had brought it up and that we could clear it up, because he had deeply cared for Michael and had been at such a loss to deal with his illness.

I felt a thousand percent better. And Ray did come back around. He flew in from California for Mike's Night (see Chapter 11), sat next to Michael the whole evening, and was one of the "roasters." He was magnificent.

Based on that incident and others I have heard from other patients and caregivers, I'm a firm believer in confronting your mate's friend who has disappointed you and asking why. I don't think this should be done in anger, but with great honesty. It should come with an admission that the friend or relative's disappearance has hurt you and your spouse deeply. That gives your friend a chance to state the reasons behind his or her disappearance and gives you both a chance to clear the air. I really believe that *it's important to forgive that friend, then, both in your heart and to his or her face.* The friends who disappoint us most are always among our closest friends. Such friendships can usually be built back again and may even be stronger for the trial they have endured.

Sometimes you simply have to accommodate someone who can't deal with your situation and understand their limitations. This is particularly true with older relatives. My father and Michael were great buddies; Dad thought the world of Michael. But whenever I called to tell him bad news about Michael, perhaps that he was in the hospital again, Dad would only say, "That's too bad. I'm real sorry, honey," and then hand the phone to my stepmother. Because she and I were very close, she told me that he would break into tears and that he didn't know what to say. He couldn't deal with the situation with me, but I knew how deeply he felt and how much he cared.

Handling Negative Feelings

If you are harboring anger or any negative feelings toward a close friend or relative who has deeply disappointed you, try the following:

1. Carefully listen to all sides of the story.
2. Put yourself in the shoes of that person and try to understand his or her motives and desperation.
3. Discuss your own feelings, opinions, and disappointments with that person.
4. Take action as appropriate in the situation.
5. If the results are still disappointing, forgive the person, make peace with yourself, and move on.

What to Do When One of Your Own Close Friends Retreats

Sometimes someone who has been a very close friend to you during your mate's chronic illness will retreat quietly and without any explanation. Suddenly you seem to be doing all the calling. They're too busy to make plans to get together or they cancel appointments once they're made. This happened four different times to me with four of my closest friends.

I couldn't share this with Michael because he had no concept of how much I depended on these people, so I started trying to figure out on my own what their reasons for backing away might be. These are the ones I came up with, and later conversations confirmed their validity.

1. They felt I was becoming too dependent on them and losing my self-confidence.
2. They could no longer deal with the situation.
3. They were going through their own personal problems and didn't want to burden me with them.
4. They cared too much. This is a particular danger with male-female friendships. The other person may begin to feel that what traditionally has been friendship-love is shading over into love-love, and he or she will back away.

Walking and jogging alone near our new home in the country was one of my needed stress-reducing activities. I vividly recall some of those times—jogging, talking aloud and weeping openly, searching desperately for answers. I was not questioning about Michael; I could not comprehend why one of my very best friends had "abandoned" me.

Usually the friend who retreats has no intention of running away or hiding forever and will come back when circumstances change. One of the four friends mentioned above, a woman in her early forties whom I had not heard from since Michael became ill, called recently to tell me that a mutual friend of ours had died unexpectedly. "I don't know what to do," she said. "I can't cope with death and dying. I've never been to a funeral. That's why I couldn't deal with Michael's illness." I told her that I believed it was up to the caregiver to decide whether to take back a friend who had backed away and that I had long ago decided to forgive her.

I would advise handling the friend who retreats much as you would the friend who disappoints. Express your feelings about the situation, forgive the person, and try to rebuild the friendship. The love and caring that were there before do not change.

We caregivers have to remember that we are a big responsibility to our true friends. Unlike our spouses, they never vowed to take us "for better or for worse."

Why You Need to Be a Good Friend

As a caregiver, being a good friend is one of the most important things you can do. Building and maintaining your own network of support will go a long way toward guaranteeing that you keep the healthy mental outlook essential to sustaining a positive attitude and being a good caregiver.

Irene is married to a diabetic who has had several strokes and has lost both his legs and much of his eyesight:

> After six years people just can't come by every week and bring food or flowers. I feel bitter that I'm out of the mainstream, and I wonder why my friends don't come by. But then I realize that they have their own lives. With a long, long illness it's hard to keep up friendships. Sometimes I feel really isolated.

Irene's plight illustrates the ironic fact that a caregiver has to work especially hard at building and maintaining friendships. That doesn't necessarily seem fair, but it's true. In the first place, you are out of the mainstream.

After a while it's easy for friends to forget to include you in their plans unless *you* take the initiative and arrange to get together with them.

From my own experience I realize that a caregiver needs to have a lot of friends, because you need your friends frequently and over a long period of time. That's really the main way I found to keep from wearing people out with my own needs. To need a lot of friends a little seemed to work better for me than to need a few friends a lot.

Miranda, whose husband has advanced lung disease, is also making a conscious effort to build up her network of support:

> One thing I've noticed lately is that I've become concerned with having enough friends. Isn't that crazy? I've never worried about having enough friends. I mean, how many is enough and how many is not enough and how many is too many? You normally don't think in terms like that. But lately I have been concerned about that and recontacting friends I haven't seen for a while and making sure we get together.
>
> I think part of it is an unconscious preparation for the time when I am alone, because Arthur has become my best friend, and he's the person I talk to all the time and the person I rely on. There's going to be a need to fill that void. I've been taking an inventory of where I stand with friends and friendships, because I have no family here.

Single adults work hard at maintaining good, true friends. If there is a possibility that you may be single again one day, it's important to work at building friendships.

Don't Be a Grouch Potato

It's an old adage that to have a friend you have to *be* a friend. This is not easy when so much of your time, attention, and energy is taken up caring for a chronically ill spouse. If you're always too busy to see your friends or even to talk to them on the phone, all but the most persistent will get discouraged and eventually drop out of sight. Once you've made time for someone, though, and you get together, your attitude and what you bring to that friendship are of paramount importance.

There were times during Michael's illness when I thought of myself as a grouch potato. At those times I didn't even like myself, so I wouldn't have blamed anyone else for not liking me either. Once I became aware of that, I realized that, while it was bad enough to be a grouch potato and know it, it was far worse to be one and *not* know it. If you know it, you can at least warn your friends, then laugh about it. But if you don't know when you're doing more than your considerable share of complaining, you can well end up making your friends as grouchy as you are— and resentful of you for doing it.

One way to be a good friend while you're also being a caregiver is to be aware of your moods. It is truly a delicate balance you must maintain to allow your friends to function as an emotional support system for you and yet to refrain from continually inflicting your day-to-day anxieties, discouragements, and frustrations on them. Knowing when you've shared enough takes practice—and a lot of sensitivity to the way your friends respond to the information you give them.

Communication works two ways. When I called friends to tell them how I was hurting, I realized I needed to be ready to listen to their problems and frustrations as well. That helps keep a friendship in balance. "You go first" are magic words to tell your friend in a conversation, regardless of who called whom. Remember to listen intently, not just wait until they take a breath so you can start! It's easy to get wrapped up in your own world, but it's really important to keep two-way communication going if you want to maintain a friendship.

I found it was a good idea, too, to contact friends now and then when I was in a good mood and everything was going well. I'd share a joke or give them a "freebie"—listen to *their* problems and frustrations without having to unload any of my own. Such calls or visits are vitally important. They keep friends from always associating you with depressing news.

After Michael died, I realized I was not calling on my friends for quite the same type or depth of support I had looked for in the past. I guess I first became aware of it four months after the funeral when I went away for a three-day weekend at a spa. I sat at dinner one evening with three strangers and we talked throughout the meal. When dinner was over, I realized it was the first time in five years I had talked so long without ever saying a word about Michael. It was truly a milestone for me. I thought to myself, "They don't even know."

The support system of friends that nurtured me so well through Michael's illness is changing quietly and almost without notice. The crisis is over now. My life is returning to normal or establishing itself into a New Normal. That is as it should be. There is no need to keep burdening people who have given me such excellent emotional support for so long with problems I can now handle on my own. Our conversations are turning back to business, people, places, and things again—surface, but interesting, topics. And yet I know now something that I did not know about myself before Michael became ill: I can always dip down into that level of feeling again when I need to, to share a crisis of my own or offer emotional support to a friend who is in need. It is an enormously comforting thing to know.

BEAR IN MIND:

You can draw reinforcement and strength from sharing events in your personal life with friends and business associates you feel close to.

Maintain a network of friends; they can make a vital contribution to a chronically ill person's quality of life. This is equally true for the caregiver.

Let friends help. As a caregiver, you are really not fine all the time. But if you don't let other people know that, they won't be able to help you.

Examine your friendships. You may find that different friends and relatives are fulfilling different functions in your life in relation to your situation with your spouse. Based on these functions, you can put friendships into categories.

Confront friends who disappear. Every patient and caregiver we talked to said there had been at least one friend who had disappointed him or her. I'm a firm believer in confronting these friends and asking them why they have disappeared from your lives in this crisis. Then I think it's important to forgive them, both in your heart and in person.

Make new friends. A caregiver needs a lot of friends because you need your friends a lot. Make time for them. Be aware of your moods around them. Remember communication works two ways, so listen to their problems, too. And share a laugh now and then.

6
Sex and
Chronic Illness

Michael was ill for half our married life. A chronic illness always affects a couple's sexual relationship on some level, and it certainly affected ours. Looking back now, I realize that I had a lot of questions I would have loved to have asked someone who was in a position to give me some answers. And yet, *even though my cousin is one of the leading sex therapists in Atlanta, it never once occurred to me to call and talk to her.*

That's how private sex can be.

All but a few of our interview subjects were reluctant to talk about their own sexual relationships, even though they were guaranteed anonymity. I am equally uncomfortable talking about mine and Michael's, protective of his privacy as well as my own. We turned instead to professionals for much of this chapter: Jeanne Shaw, Ph.D., a certified sex therapist and clinical psychologist with a nursing background; Bill Talmadge, Ph.D., a psychologist who includes sex therapy as part of his practice and counsels a number of couples in which one partner is chronically ill; and Sally Lehr, R.N., M.N., a clinical specialist in psychiatric mental health nursing who teaches the course "Human Sexuality in Health and Illness" at the Emory University School of Nursing in Atlanta.

How Chronic Illness Affects a Couple's Sexuality

"When people get ill they think sex isn't part of the 'sick' role," says Sally Lehr. "Sometimes the spouses of the ill persons are afraid they are going to do something to hurt their mates, or they feel guilty for even wanting a sexual relationship."

Too often both parties keep silent about the situation. For many of us, it's a "solution" dictated by our upbringing. Many of us were raised to believe that you simply didn't talk about sex—not with *anybody.* For those of us in our forties or older, such an upbringing was virtually universal.

Illnesses such as diabetes or multiple sclerosis can affect a man's ability to have an erection. This can play havoc with a man's self-esteem—and with his wife's as well, if she mistakenly assumes that the situation reflects her husband's feelings toward her.

Many drugs also can affect sexual performance. In men they can affect the ability to get or keep an erection. In women, their effect is experienced more as a general lessening of the desire for sex. The *Physician's Desk Reference* lists every prescription drug available in the United States, tells what it is prescribed for, and gives suggested dosages and possible side effects. The book is available in the reference room of any library. Since it is updated annually, one- or two-year-old editions can often be purchased cheaply at used bookstores. Several similar books, aimed not at physicians but at lay readers, can also be found in libraries and bookstores. If you and your spouse think your sexual problems may be due to a prescription drug, you might want to check out the possible side effects in the *Physician's Desk Reference* or a similar publication and then talk to your doctor about the situation. The problem can often be solved by changing medication or dosage.

Extreme weight gain or weight loss, the presence of a scar, and the absence of a limb can all deal leaden blows to self-image and make a patient reluctant to initiate sex.

Carol, like many others, blows up like a balloon from steroid therapy:

> It's very difficult to have a real good image of your body when you know that in the last month you've gained eighteen pounds. You see yourself in the mirror and your eyes are swollen and your waist has increased in size four or five inches and every day of your life you feel horrible. You lose perspective on your sexuality. You don't feel sexually attractive to yourself or believe that you could be to your spouse.

Sometimes blows to the patient's self-image are not immediately recognizable for what they are. Elaine's husband had a problem after a bout with colon cancer:

> He felt that I was not affectionate to him and found him unattractive because his operation left a scar, even though I told him it didn't bother me. I think he attributed to me a lot of the things he didn't want to feel himself. He would say, "You feel this" and "You feel that," when in fact he was the one who felt it.

Just because your spouse is chronically ill, however, does not automatically mean that your sexual relationship has to suffer. Dr. Shaw tells of a couple she counseled who dissolve into giggles every time they talk about making love. She lacks the use of her arms; he is a paraplegic, paralyzed from the waist down. Just getting into bed is a major accomplishment in itself, and the actual act of making love is even more complicated for this determined couple. But here are two people who are living proof that where there's a will there's a way. They have turned what many others might have taken as insurmountable obstacles into a series of hilarious challenges that produce a rich experience of joy for the two of them.

For many couples where a chronic and limiting medical condition is present, however, the course of true love—and sexual interaction—does not run so smoothly.

What Sexual Relationship?

Many aspects of chronic illness can adversely affect a couple's sex life:

- *Physiological problems.* Illnesses such as diabetes or multiple sclerosis can make it difficult for a man to sustain an erection.
- *Stamina.* Chronic illness can sap energy that would ordinarily go into maintaining a sexual relationship.
- *Drugs.* Many prescription drugs can affect sexual performance. If you think this is happening, check with your doctor. Often a prescription can be changed.
- *Self-image.* Dramatic weight gain or weight loss, a new scar, or the loss of a limb may make the patient feel he or she is no longer sexually attractive.
- *The "sick role."* Often the care-giving spouse assumes that because his or her partner is ill it would be inappropriate to suggest having sex.
- *The stress of caregiving.* When taking care of your spouse takes up a lot of your time, you may temporarily cease thinking about having sex.

"The stress of a chronic medical condition is going to show up any cracks in a marriage," says Dr. Talmadge, "any problems that were already there. In terms of sex, what you may see is a breakdown in the affection in the relationship. The well person may begin to interpret the other person's illness as a personal rejection."

The caregiver may simply cease to see the ill spouse as sexual, he says, particularly when the caregiving has come to take up a considerable portion of their life together. "That's only natural, and people need to understand that," he says. "It doesn't mean you've ceased to look upon that person as your love object. When you see your wife laid up in the hospital after surgery, you don't want to have sex with her. You want to take care of her and make her feel better."

Sometimes, however, particularly when they don't talk openly about the fact that sex seems to have disappeared from their marital relationship, a couple may find themselves growing distant from one another. One person may stay up much later than the other as a way of avoiding sex. The couple may find they hardly talk to one another, not just intimate conversation, but conversation of any kind. Signs of affection—hand-holding, kissing, caressing, saying "I love you"—may have disappeared as well. When these things happen, that's the time to go for help.

Where to Get Help

The doctor is the first person many couples turn to for help. Sometimes he or she can answer your questions, particularly if the sexual problems involved are physiological. Often, however, your physician cannot provide you with the information you need. Until the mid-1970s, few medical schools offered courses in human sexuality.

It's important to remember that doctors are human beings, too. Like many of the rest of us, they may feel uncomfortable when confronted with issues involving sexuality. Katy, who has suffered from severe and life-threatening asthma since childhood, tells of her experience with her doctor when she had a permanent IV implanted under the skin on her breast, a procedure she hoped would cut down on hospital visits:

> It had to be attached to a rib and connected to a vein close to the heart. The doctors thought I was crazy when I said, "I am going to tell you how I want this put, because my husband holds my boobs when I go to sleep at night. The last thing he needs is a great hunk of metal in the middle." So I told them where to put it, and they thought it was hilarious. I didn't. You

have to take charge at times, because your doctors don't think about sexuality and they don't want to talk about it, either.

If you do consult your physician, follow the guidelines in Chapter 12. Notify him or her in advance about what you want to discuss and say that you might need a little extra time. Ask honest and direct questions—it helps to write them down beforehand so you won't forget anything. If your doctor tries to dismiss your questions about sex, ask where you can go to get the help you need. He or she may give you the name of a psychologist or a sex therapist in private practice, or you might be referred to a counseling center maintained by a church or a community mental health center. These facilities often operate on a sliding fee scale based on ability to pay.

You can also do a lot on your own, say the professionals, toward maintaining a healthy sexual relationship with a chronically ill spouse. The most important thing you can do is keep the lines of communication open. That means talking together about any sexual problems you might have.

Why Talk About Sex?

One goal of therapy with couples is always to improve communication between the partners—about the sexual relationship and the marriage in general. "Sex issues are almost always more than just sex issues," says Dr. Shaw.

A study by psychologist Helen Frank appeared several years ago in the *New England Journal of Medicine*. When Dr. Frank compared fifty couples who were in therapy with fifty couples who were not, she found virtually the same number of sexually dysfunctional couples in each group. She concluded that the major difference between the couples who had gone into therapy and the couples who hadn't was that the couples in the latter group were able to talk about their sexual difficulties with each other.

When something goes wrong with any couple's sexual relationship, the most important thing the partners can do is discuss it. This is particularly true when one partner is chronically ill. Illness complicates any situation. As a caregiver, you cannot know everything your ill spouse is feeling. The stress and pain of chronic illness makes your partner less conscious of your needs and feelings than he or she would be otherwise.

In most situations, the ill person is the one whose sexuality is most affected. But the stress of caregiving, or changes in the ill patient, can affect the caregiver's sexuality, too. *Sometimes neither person says anything about the fact that sex is disappearing from the marriage.* The patient, who feels inadequate to provide it, doesn't want to broach the subject. The spouse doesn't want to bring it up for fear of putting an extra burden on the patient or hurting his or her feelings. Although the mutual silence may indicate that both partners have accepted the new nonsexual relationship, many unspoken questions still hang in the air.

"Not talking about an issue that comes up in a marriage, particularly a sexual issue, creates distance between the couple," says Dr. Shaw. "It builds a wall that can result in resentment or depression for the patient and the caregiver." A second reason for talking about your sexual needs and feelings with your ill spouse, she adds, is that by not doing so you depersonalize and diminish your spouse:

> We tend to diminish disabled people by thinking they can't do things for themselves—and I'm not just talking about physical things. I'm talking about protecting the patient against something *you* think might be unpleasant for him or her without giving the patient the chance to decide whether it's unpleasant or not.

If there are *aspects* of sex, such as the ability to have intercourse, that are lost due to chronic illness, it is normal for both the ill husband or wife and the care-giving spouse to feel grief, just as they do for other aspects of health and independence that have been lost. Reminiscing about the way sex used to be and talking about what has been lost, says Dr. Shaw, give the couple the chance to grieve together. This can help bridge any distance that has grown between them and bring them closer to one another.

She tells of a young couple who were in an auto accident. The husband was driving the car and sustained only slight injuries. The wife was left paralyzed from the neck down. After ten bitter years their marriage ended in divorce. "The problem was they had never grieved about the accident together," she says. "They refused to be sad with each other and cry and talk about their losses. All of this was like a wound that was abscessed way down deep, and every time anybody touched the top of it, it hurt all the way down.

"If he's alone in his anguish and she's alone in her anguish," Dr. Shaw continues, "then that's twice as much anguish. Two people get some relief when they can grieve together. It takes away the uniqueness and the loneliness of it and makes the grieving a 'couples' thing to do."

How to Talk to Each Other About Sex

Many partners aren't comfortable talking to each other about their sexual relationship even under the best of circumstances. Dr. Shaw tells a poignant yet all too typical story of a couple she counseled. In separate conversations with husband and wife, it emerged that for the entire twenty years of their marriage the husband had blown in his wife's ear as a prelude to lovemaking, thinking that was the thing that most excited her—and for the entire twenty years she had hated it because it reminded her of the earaches she'd had as a child. Yet throughout all this time she had never admitted she didn't like it for fear of hurting her husband's feelings.

"A couple's sexual needs, wants, and desires—or what they don't want, what they don't like, and what they wish their partners wouldn't do—it's all kind of a sticky subject to begin with," says Dr. Shaw. Add to this normal reluctance the complications of a chronic illness, and the subject becomes even harder to approach.

There is no easy formula for initiating a discussion about sex with your chronically ill spouse. The professionals we interviewed did, however, offer a few pointers. Dr. Talmadge suggests reading something together about chronic illness and its impact on sexuality:

> I've found that to be very helpful, particularly for the partner who doesn't have the illness. It helps them externalize the illness, instead of taking the ill partner's loss of sexual function as a personal rejection. The man may have difficulty getting an erection because he has multiple sclerosis, for example, but the wife thinks it's because he isn't attracted to her anymore. If they read something together that says multiple sclerosis can interfere with a man's ability to get an erection, they can talk about their situation and their feelings about it and she'll be reassured.

Dr. Talmadge mentions in particular a publication put out by the National Multiple Sclerosis Society, *About Sexuality and People with Disabilities,* and another by the Arthritis Foundation entitled *Arthritis, Living and Loving, Information About Sex.* A number of books on particular illnesses contain chapters on sexuality. "It is important that both partners read the information," Dr. Talmadge stresses, "and it's best that they read it together, that they do this as a couple."

Sally Lehr suggests initiating a conversation about sex by first acknowledging that it is something you feel uncomfortable talking about. "If you say something like, 'This is really uncomfortable for me to talk about, but sex has been such an important part of our marriage in the past that I feel like I need to talk about it now with you in spite of that,' then that helps to break the tension," she advises. "Acknowledge that you don't have all the answers but are willing to talk about it because it's something you're concerned about."

She also suggests reading on the subject and then using that reading to put your situation into a larger context:

> If you say something like, "I've been reading that people in our situation often experience a decrease in sexual desire for each other," that lets the other partner know that it's OK to talk about sex and that there are a lot of other people out there in the same boat as you two. I use similar techniques in teaching my nursing students how to interview their patients about sexual concerns, and not one of them has reported having a bad experience.

How to Talk to Your Spouse About Sex

- Appoint a specific time to talk about your sexual relationship when you know you won't be disturbed. Say what it is you are going to talk about, then *talk* about it.
- Read some information *together* on the impact of chronic illness on sexuality. Not only will this give you something to discuss, it will let you know there are other people in the same situation as you.
- Admit that talking about your sexual relationship makes you uncomfortable and that you don't have all the answers, but that sex is important enough to you that you feel the need to discuss it anyway.
- Express your feelings openly and honestly. Admit, for example, that you're sad because you miss the kind of sexual relationship the two of you used to have or that you're angry because you loved the way the two of you made love before the illness. Talking about feelings like these helps clear the air.
- If your partner categorically refuses to talk with you about your sexual relationship, try talking about it to a trusted friend.

Dr. Shaw suggests talking openly and honestly about the fact that you miss the sexual relationship you used to have:

> If a couple can talk about what they miss, then that's a way of being close. If they can talk about their feelings about missing that particular aspect of their sexuality, then they get a chance to express feelings they've been withholding from each other, feelings like, "I'm depressed because you aren't able to do this anymore," or "I'm angry because I can't do that anymore; it was such an important part of my life and I feel like I'm cheating you out of something. I want you to know that I'm angry about it because I loved the way we had sex before." To get out feelings like that helps clear the air and make a subject that was taboo OK to talk about.

She advises the partners to appoint a specific time to talk about their sexual relationship, a time that is convenient for both of them and one when they will not be disturbed by phone calls, children, or whatever. "Second, you can say what you're going to talk about and admit that you are uncomfortable with the subject. Then the third thing is to talk about it."

In a few cases, she admits, a couple simply isn't communicating well enough in their marriage to talk about sex together. "I know some couples who, when one partner says to the other, 'I want to talk to you about something that's really important to me but I'm very uncomfortable talking about it,' the other partner just says, 'Well, if you're uncomfortable talking about it, I sure as heck don't want to hear about it.'"

Her advice in that situation is to vent your frustrations about your sexual relationship to a trusted friend. At least that way *you* will get the chance to let out your feelings.

Exploring New Options

The most powerful human sexual organ is located between the ears. We create our sexuality in our minds, but unfortunately many of us have a very narrow idea of what sex is. "People have to understand that sex is much more than just vaginal-penile intercourse," says Dr. Talmadge. "Sex occurs much more often in our heads and in our hearts and in our skin through touch. Very little occurs genitally; that's only the beginning. Helping folks to understand that can open up other avenues."

A chronic illness that may take away a couple's primary way of having sex can actually have a positive impact on the couple's sex life by encouraging them to explore other options. Sally Lehr tells of one couple she counseled: "One day the male partner came in and said, 'I had the best sex I ever had the other night, and we never had intercourse.' Changing your mindset can be an enormous adventure, and you can learn a lot about yourself and your partner."

The first thing you might have to change is any idea you cherish that the only good sex is spontaneous sex. When a chronic illness is present, good sex is more often than not the result of careful planning. Pain, loss of energy, stiffness, tiredness, and other symptoms place constraints on when and how often the ill spouse can have sex. There are ways, says Dr. Talmadge, that most people can get around them:

> It's important for the well partner to help the ill partner regulate himself or herself. If lack of stamina is a problem, help see to it that your spouse doesn't overdo on the day you plan to have sex. If chronic back pain is a problem, remind your spouse not to bend over the sink or do taxing lifting on the day the two of you have planned a romantic evening. There is often a tendency for the ill spouse to overdo as a means of denying the presence of the illness.

Encouraging your ill husband or wife at all times to take care of themselves and pace themselves is a loving and supportive thing to do. Such pacing can have particular benefits where your sexual relationship is concerned. If tiredness and loss of energy are problems, have sex at a time when your spouse is rested, which may be in the morning or the afternoon rather than at night. If pain is a problem, pain medication can be taken so that its maximum effect will coincide with when you plan to make love.

Sally Lehr also agrees that when one person is chronically ill, the first key to successful sex is good timing. "Some people think that if you have to plan it, it isn't any good," she says, "but if you have the right mindset, planning can make it even better because you have all day to look forward to it."

Tips for Good Timing

When one of the partners is ill, the secret to good sex is often good timing. Some suggestions:

- Plan in advance for lovemaking if your spouse needs to rest or otherwise prepare. Remember, anticipation can be at least as big a turn-on as spontaneity.
- If stamina is a problem, make love when your spouse is rested—in the morning or afternoon.
- Encourage your spouse not to work too hard or otherwise overdo on the day you are planning a romantic evening.
- If your spouse is on pain medication, time the taking of it so that the maximum effect will come at the time you plan to make love.

A lot of people give up on being sexual when intercourse is no longer possible. That, say the therapists, is a downright sad and silly thing to do. According to Dr. Shaw, "*A crisis occurs only when a person doesn't see the options.*" In sex, intercourse is only one possibility: "If two people are not disabled, they have lots of options. If one person is disabled, only one option is removed."

Often when a couple visits a therapist because of sexual problems, the therapist will forbid intercourse for a specified period of time so they will realize that there are numerous other ways of making love. "When you put a ban on intercourse, the couple is forced to start all over again in a dating situation, to learn to touch each other all over again, to learn what feels good to each other," says Sally Lehr. "It's a kind of reeducation, learning that other activities are really nice."

It isn't always easy. Learning how to touch and be touched can be particularly difficult for some men. Many men grow up never really knowing how to touch people and not really being responsive to touch. Learning that touching really feels nice can be a whole new thing for them.

You might find it helpful to have some idea of what is possible. Dr. Shaw offers a partial list:

> The two of you can talk about sex together, have sexual fantasies together, talk about how good sex used to be, or stimulate each other sexually with your hands or with your mouths. You can masturbate or hold your partner while he or she masturbates. There are a lot of sexual options that many people just don't know about or don't exercise, either because they're too embarrassed or because mother said, "Nice people don't do that."
>
> Persons with physical disabilities often discover they have erotic areas on their bodies that other people don't even think of, like the backs of the knees, the ankles, the toes, the ears, the neck. Persons who are paralyzed with spinal cord injuries, for example, become exquisitely sensitive in the skin that has sensual perception left.

To help you learn more about your sexual options, a good marriage manual can prove invaluable. You will find such books in the psychology section or the sex and marriage section of your local bookstore. Buy one, take it home—and read it together. Remember, the goal of making love is nothing more—and nothing less—than that the two of you enjoy it.

Exploring Your Sexual Options

When a couple is having sexual difficulties and seeks professional help, often the first thing the therapist does is put a ban on intercourse for a period of time. This makes the couple feel freer than they ordinarily might to explore the other sexual options available to them. Often chronic illness puts its own ban on intercourse. The following are some other ways you might choose to express your sexuality to one another:

- Talk about sex together, including how good sex used to be.
- Share a sexual fantasy—what would you like to do together if you could do anything you wanted?
- Kiss, cuddle, and caress.
- Try touching each other in new places. As the result of illness or disability, some people may become exquisitely sensitive in places other people don't even think of as erotic, such as behind the knees or on the palms of the hands or on the neck.
- Bring your spouse to orgasm with your hand or with your mouth.
- Bring yourself to orgasm in your spouse's presence while he or she holds you or hold your spouse while he or she does the same.

Consult a good marriage manual to learn of still more things the two of you can do.

Relationships Outside the Marriage

Sometimes when chronic illness puts its stress on a marriage, one of the partners will decide to go outside the marriage for sex. While not endorsing this, therapists admit that on occasion such a move can be the salvation of the marital union. Most advise caregivers who are considering an affair to get professional help first. Such therapy will at least enable them to sort out the motives behind such a drastic move and understand how such an action can be reconciled with the feelings they have for their spouse.

While this is excellent advice, I fear it is generally advice not taken. As romantic literature tells us time and again, an affair most often begins as a sexually and emotionally charged event and rarely as a conscious decision. Even when it does, it's not a decision participants tend to think through; *they do not want to know the ramifications their actions may have.*

Most often a person thinking about entering into an affair, if he or she does discuss their decision with someone else, will go to a friend or to their minister or other spiritual advisor. In either case they are likely to know what the reaction will be. Their spiritual leader will attempt to dissuade them; their friend will most likely stand by them. Which person they choose to confide in is a valuable clue to the answer they are seeking—and to the decision they have probably already made.

There can be numerous reasons for seeking a sexual relationship outside the marriage when a chronic illness is involved. "Sometimes an affair is a symptom of emotional withdrawal, feeling like you want to get away from the illness or deny it," says Sally Lehr. Some patients recognize the presence of this denial in their spouses and admit to being more permissive regarding their spouse's sexual conduct than they would ordinarily be. On occasion, says, Sally Lehr, it's the patient who has the affair: "Sometimes sick people put themselves in other relationships as a way of denying their illness."

Dr. Shaw recommends renegotiating the marriage when a spouse wants to have an affair: discussing the situation and setting up rules for the affair, such as no emotional involvement. Such renegotiation may actually help keep some marriages together in the long run. What hurts is when one person has sex outside the marriage in anger, as a way of expressing anger toward the marriage partner. It hurts because the air hasn't been cleared by bringing it out into the open.

If the relationship is renegotiated into a nonsexual marriage, Dr. Shaw points out, this can actually empower the patient because suddenly he or she has something to give:

> Generally, the person who's physically ill will feel like a burden being catered to and waited on. He or she can't go out and work, help with the housework, or otherwise pull any weight in the family. How can this person feel less burdensome? One way is to rethink the marriage vows. Yes, it's a burden to keep your partner celibate, but you can unburden yourself and your partner from the sexual responsibility by giving your partner permission to find that someplace else.

Sometimes the caregiver may get into a fairly serious relationship outside marriage that is not sexual. Vanessa's husband suffered a stroke in his early thirties that robbed him of his ability to work and of some of his intellectual capacity. She admits to having entered into several "intense intellectual friendships" with male colleagues to fill the void:

> There were times when I was incredibly lonely for healthy, male companionship. I was lonely for somebody with good biceps to go hiking the Appalachian trail with or for someone who could carry our child around in a backpack and go all day someplace. I wound up seeking out a few men in a work context in a fairly obsessive way. There was never any remote progression toward an affair, but they fulfilled at least some of my needs.

For Vanessa, these nonsexual relationships were enough.

The Long Haul

Chronic illness presents enormous challenges to a marital relationship, but they are challenges couples can, and do, overcome. Some couples do it instinctively, the way Michael and I maintained our closeness by continuing to touch, show each other affection and respect, and talk together about how much we still loved each other. Other couples are helped by professional guidance. What it all comes down to is a realization that sexuality can take many forms. It can be reaching over to touch a hand or stroke a head. It can be giving a backrub. Sex isn't only what the therapists term "penis and vagina" intercourse; sex is a continuum—and you can enjoy it anywhere along the way. "A couple's desire to stay together, even through this kind of a trial, is the biggest factor in keeping that love alive," says Dr. Talmadge.

When Jesse and Pam first married, she was "this hot-blooded Italian lady who would get in the shower when I was in there and drop her drawers." In the early years of their marriage, however, Pam developed severe heart problems and has since had several strokes. They continued their sexual relationship, although in the beginning Jesse's greatest fear was that she would have a heart attack and die during sex. Pam decided that the risk was worth it, and Jesse decided he could live with that:

> The only advice I would give anybody about sex is that you both be in accord on what you want to do and that you both maintain a sensitivity to each other's wants and needs. I think that takes care of it all. If you're sensitive to her condition and she's sensitive to yours, that puts just as much pressure on her as it does on you. If you're both sensitive to each other and you know you want to work something out, then you normally work it out. The most important thing is that both parties realize there will be a change in their relationship, but that doesn't mean avoiding

sex. You'd be surprised what you can do when you set your mind to it. We've hardly missed a beat—in all these years.

BEAR IN MIND:

Remember that certain illnesses—and many drugs—can affect a man's ability to have an erection.

Look for creative ways to please each other. Just because your spouse is chronically ill does not automatically mean that your sexual relationship has to suffer.

Look for a doctor with whom you can discuss your feelings. Even many doctors feel uncomfortable when confronted with issues involving sexuality.

Maintain open communications. Sometimes neither person says anything about the fact that sex is disappearing from the marriage.

Expand your ideas about what sex is. The most powerful human sexual organ is located between the ears.

Plan ahead. When chronic illness is present, good sex is more often than not the result of careful planning.

Explore. Persons with physical disabilities often discover they have erotic areas that other people don't even think of.

7
Vacations, Travel, Holidays, and Hobbies

The most recent crisis is now over, and life settles into its New Normal. You become immersed in your daily routine, but your husband or wife begins to get restless and bored. What is there to do?

One of you boldly suggests, "Why don't we go somewhere?" You go through some quick mental gymnastics as you think of the oxygen tank, the wheelchair or crutches, and of the anxiety of putting added mileage between you and the medical team. The obstacles seem insurmountable, but so does the thought of hanging around the house for another twenty or thirty years. You reconsider: perhaps you can't do everything you had planned before, but can't you substitute new dreams for the ones that are no longer possible?

Using Ingenuity to Overcome Obstacles

The vacation site that was most important to Michael and me was Grand Cayman, a scrubby little island in the British West Indies. It had no televisions or golf courses and few residential telephones. There was nothing to do, which is the very reason we loved it. Our mere arrival gave us renewed strength; the moment we stepped off the plane we felt different. Even the antiquated transportation system that took forever to bring us to our place was part of the fun.

Michael was at his best in Cayman. He was no longer the powerful executive who shouted at people and threw pencils like darts into the ceiling over his desk. Instead he became a beach bum dressed in a baggy bathing suit with a carefully selected, torn T-shirt worn inside out. He snorkeled for hours in the crystal clear waters searching for conchs, and we often found him aground on a coral reef in our dilapidated old boat with that torn T-shirt flapping from a fishing pole, signalling for help.

Our life in Cayman represented a brief spell of stability in our otherwise unpredictable lives. We continued going there throughout most of Michael's illness, and we discovered that creativity and ingenuity overcame many of the obstacles that could otherwise have made our favorite travel destination inaccessible.

The first trip back after the amputation was a touchy, delicate time. Mike was understandably self-conscious about his prosthesis, and he wore long-legged pants on the beach, even in the full heat of the Caribbean sun. Getting him into the water seemed impossible at first, but after numerous aborted attempts we hatched a daring plan. We wrapped a small swim ladder with towels and secured it to the stern of our old boat, and we went out to a shallow, protected area that was free of potential onlookers. Pretending to be Mike, I flopped over the side of the boat and into the water. I then tried to get out again, using only my upper body and one leg. Balance was tough, but I eventually worked out the most efficient routine for getting up the ladder. Mike watched and mentally rehearsed the maneuver until each move was clear in his mind so he wouldn't have to waste any strength in futile attempts. Our efforts paid off, and he was able to clamber back into the boat on the first try. It was never easy for him, but the swimming and snorkeling made the awkward reentry into the boat worthwhile.

Another favorite Cayman pastime of his was solitary

fishing. Because of his disability and his history of getting stuck on reefs, we came up with a simple idea to ensure his safety. At Radio Shack we bought a pair of inexpensive walkie-talkies designed for kids. I kept one on the porch with the volume up full blast (so neighbors could also hear), and he took one on the boat. He loved having that walkie-talkie to play with and liked the independence it gave him. It also afforded the kids and me some degree of peace. His renewed confidence and mobility came in handy one breezy day when one of the boys and a friend were out practicing for a sailboat race. Their sail split in a gust, the boat capsized, and kids and boat began drifting toward a deserted mangrove swamp. It was Mike in his trusty old boat who found them.

Planning, Planning, Planning

Traveling does not necessarily become an impossibility when your spouse is sick or disabled. It is more complicated to arrange, but many hurdles can be overcome with advance planning. Jesse continues to travel with his wife, who has endured multiple strokes:

> We learn to go at our speed, not the speed of the other tourists. Although I never check any luggage when I travel alone, when we travel together we check everything. And I always get hold of a copy of the flight schedule so I'm familiar with our options to return early in case she gets sick.

The best place to begin your adventure is with a good travel agent. Whether you are seeking a trip by air, rail, or ship, a good agent can save you time and frustration by handling much of the detail work. Tell your agent how mobile your spouse is and what kind of equipment must be brought along or provided, and let him or her pave the way for you.

Michael and I were invited to a conference in London.

Even though he was an amputee and in constant pain from his remaining leg, we badly wanted to take the trip. The mental stimulation would be important to us both, and the subject of the conference—financial planning—was relevant to our interest in providing for the future. The logistics of the trip seemed a big hurdle until our travel agent helped us out. He reserved us bulkhead seats that gave Mike maximum leg room. When we got on the plane it wasn't full, so I staked my claim to an empty row of seats. It paid to be aggressive—Mike could go back, stretch out, and elevate his leg whenever necessary.

Our agent also helped us select a postconference trip that enabled us to see some European countryside without doing any walking. We chose a three-day boat trip down the Rhine River in Germany. At each landing Michael decided whether or not he felt up to a land excursion in his wheelchair; if he did not, he encouraged me to go without him. On the advice of our agent we never attempted organized bus tours but instead hired a taxi and saw the sights at our own pace.

If you search diligently, you may be lucky enough to find a tour arranged especially for people with your spouse's type of illness. "Traveling is a darn nuisance, and I haven't done much of it since I began using oxygen," said Kelly a year ago. Like forty-seven million other Americans who suffer from some form of pulmonary disease, she thought she was destined to spend the rest of her life at home. Then she heard about a company in Atlanta called Glasrock Home Health Care, which had an organized tour for people with breathing problems. Suddenly Kelly found herself able to take the trip of a lifetime, a cruise to the Caribbean.

Glasrock handled all the details of the trip. They asked Kelly to get travel permission from her physician and required her to pass certain rehabilitation programs. Next they compiled information to show the cruise line that oxygen equipment is safe and reliable and does not pose a hazard to other passengers. They arranged for an oxygen supply company to provide equipment for the ship and training sessions on its handling. They also made special arrangements with the airline for the use of portable oxygen equipment during the flight to the cruise ship's port of embarkation. They even arranged special ground transportation.

Complicated? Yes. Doable? Yes. Worth it? Absolutely. Glasrock is hopeful that its efforts will break the ice for other disabled people and help the travel industry realize that reliance upon life-support equipment shouldn't prevent anyone from leaving home.

Glasrock is not the only group that helps the physically handicapped continue to travel. The Society for the Advancement of Travel for the Handicapped helps travel agencies make arrangements for accommodations to suit disabled persons. Many of the large hotel and motel chains have directories listing the handicapped-accessible facilities at their various locations. Mobility International in London, which has offices throughout Europe, provides information and even has an exchange program.

Did you know that all of the major car rental agencies have cars equipped with hand controls? That the major bus lines allow a handicapped traveler and a companion to travel together on one ticket? That Amtrak provides a free brochure on its services for elderly and handicapped passengers? That other organizations publish pamphlets on subjects such as safe boating for the handicapped and airport terminal accessibility? That there are wheelchair bowling leagues, motorcycle clubs, and pilots associations? That there are a deaf skiers organization and an association for blind athletes? That Outward Bound has outdoor adventure programs for the disabled? That the National Park Service offers a lifetime passport to the handicapped that admits them—and any others traveling in the same car— for half price?

The world is waiting. All you have to do is tap into the many resources available to help you learn how to get about. And if you stumble into a less-than-cooperative person or two, don't be discouraged. All of the paraphernalia our traveling buddies need, for instance, can be a logistical headache. Oxygen equipment in particular presents an obstacle that many people don't realize can be overcome. The airlines vary in their cooperativeness, so it pays to shop around. Some refuse to handle oxygen equipment, while others will provide it for a nominal charge if you can show a letter from your doctor. Your local supplier can often help relieve some of the hassle by arranging to have equipment waiting for you at the other end of your flight.

Don't be put off by an initial negative response to your request for special consideration. Many employees are simply ignorant about what is possible, and even management personnel sometimes need help in opening their eyes to unusual situations. "I have educated a lot of airline employees over the last few years on the fact that yes, they can supply in-flight oxygen, and here's how it works," says one caregiver who refuses to leave his wife behind when he travels. Go straight to the top if that's what it takes to open doors or change company policy.

Don't Wait Until . . .

There are many stories of couples who are waiting to travel until . . . until the kids grow up . . . until we retire . . . until we can afford to do it right. Then illness strikes and a twenty-year dream disintegrates. How many times have you heard people moan that they wish they had traveled more when they could?

In spite of the pain Michael was in during our wonderful trip to London and Germany, we never doubted that it was the right thing to do. The day we returned to the United States he went straight to the hospital and four weeks later lost his other leg. We were both happy that we had not waited "until he felt better" to take that trip, because if we had he would have ended up feeling depressed and deprived. Instead he was filled with happy memories that helped him through the trying weeks ahead.

Don't put off that trip you've got your heart set on. With spunk and determination it is possible that you can still go. Vicki and Brad were determined to keep on traveling even after Brad had several strokes and was transformed from a busy executive into a bored house husband:

> We both had an incredible urge to travel but we had always said, "We'll do it later." After his illness began we knew we had to do it now. I took every day of vacation I had. During the past twelve years we have been to Mexico, Greece, Israel, Egypt, the Soviet Union, and China. We just came back from France. *This was our gift to ourselves.* It has given us something to look forward to and work for and has helped take away some of the "Why did this have to happen to us?"

These trips weren't crisis-free, but so far no problem has been insurmountable:

> One time in Italy Brad was sick as a goat, but I was able to leave him to rest in the hotel room. Another time I had to take him off a cruise ship in Acapulco because we had used up every bit of oxygen on the ship, but after four days in the Marriott I got him on his feet and back home again. Once Brad said, "Vicki, if I drop dead in France it will be no more difficult than if I drop dead at home." I said, "Yes it will, because I would still have to get you back. I don't know how to do that!" We were able to laugh about it.

In order to afford yourselves of the best medical care should things go wrong on a trip, you might ask your doctor ahead of time to supply you with names of specialists in the countries or cities you plan to visit. If that doesn't work, the International Association for Medical Assistance to Travellers has a brochure that lists English-speaking physicians all over the world. It can be obtained by writing them at 736 Centre Street, Lewiston, New York 14092, or by phoning (716) 754-4883.

Take That Chance

At the beginning of an illness everything can seem so new and unknown that the mere thought of travel is frightening. Once the initial crisis is passed, however, and you settle into your new routines and become more comfortable with your changed circumstances, adventurous feelings may emerge. When Amy was first diagnosed with lupus her world was turned upside down. Now, only a year later, she is ready to take the risk of getting out of the house:

> I'm thinking of taking the kids on a camping trip to Death Valley and the national parks. My husband can't take time off work so I'm going to take them myself. What happens if I wake up and I'm not having such a good day? I'll take that chance. Last fall I would never have thought of going that far from home. It takes a little while to know what to expect, but now I have more of a sense of what the parameters are in terms of ups and downs.

Understanding the new and constantly changing parameters does not mean, "Here's what you cannot do"; it means, "Now we can determine what is possible." This allows someone like Amy to set her sights on more distant horizons:

> Even now we're thinking about what we're going to do next summer. We'd like to go to Europe. I don't know if I will be well or off the medication, and that adds complexity and some insecurity. But if we stay in a place that is comfortable, I can rest for an afternoon while Lewis takes the kids out.

Vacations and holidays are what most people look forward to fifty weeks of the year. For the disabled, handicapped, or ill person, those dreams must not be crushed. Today's travel and exploration possibilities are limited only by our imaginations. Charlie is a paraplegic confined to a wheelchair for life. He lives in a small southern town that has one scuba shop with a sign outside that says, "Learn to dive." Each time he passed that sign Charlie yearned to feel warm, tropical water around his imprisoned body, but he was discouraged by the comments his family made. One day he rebelled. He insisted that they stop and ask the shop owner to come outside to talk with him. "I want to learn to dive," he said. The shop owner replied, without a moment's hesitation, "Classes start next Saturday. If you have the will to dive, I can teach you." Charlie took the course, passed the pool and classroom tests, and became a certified diver on his open water dive in Cozumel, Mexico.

Too often we settle for simply *wishing* we could do something, without making any attempts to turn our dreams into reality. If you and your spouse have the will to travel, explore those dreams! Make them a reality!

Ready . . . Set . . . Go!

You have established a New Normal in your lives. You both have gotten used to (well, maybe not used to, but you can deal with it) the embarrassment of being stared at in public, the effort and the hassle to get out. You are pumped up and ready to pack your bags and medical equipment and get on with life. What now? What are some of your travel options, and how do you find out about them?

You may need to challenge your travel agency. "There are some unique, special kinds of tours that someone in a wheelchair or with some degree of impairment would find delightful," says my agent, who gives the example of luxury coach tours offered on the West Coast. The buses are equipped with oversized captain's chairs for extra comfort, VCRs to brief guests on upcoming attractions, microwave ovens for the preparation of special dietary requirements, and stereos to provide music along the way. What a great way to see the coast of California!

Your agent should have a multitude of ideas to choose from. Another option is to plan things yourself, contacting cruise lines, railroads, or the airlines directly. Better still, let your spouse plan the trip. You provide a telephone, some current travel magazines, the travel section from the Sunday paper, and a big tablet on which to make notes. Let him or her enjoy the challenge and fun of planning the trip. Vicki has found this to be a useful tactic for her husband:

> Brad has the responsibility and activity of planning the trip, studying the geography and history of the destination, and reading about it for many months. This has really been a boost to his morale, and it gives him something to discuss with the people he sees.

Whether your travel dreams must be limited to a place near home or faraway lands are your next destination, a zillion questions must be answered before you decide on specifics. If you are going on a cruise, for example, be sure your ship pulls into a dock rather than anchoring in the harbor and ferrying passengers ashore, because when you have equipment to drag along with you those little boats can be an insurmountable obstacle. If you are bringing special equipment, contact the medical officer or the captain in advance. Ship policy will probably require that the patient be traveling with an able-bodied person and that you sign a release to protect the ship from liability.

One good resource for ideas and specific information is your local library or bookstore. Just one example of the treasures to be found there is a book called *Access America: An Atlas and Guide for Visitors with Disabilities*, which gives details on thirty-seven national parks.

You may both enjoy exploring new places, but on your first trip from home you might prefer the security of going back to a place you enjoyed in the past. This enables you to mentally walk through each activity—arriving, settling into the room, negotiating restaurants, and so on—to spot most problems before they are actually encountered. *I have often found visualization to be a positive technique for working out logistics well ahead of time.*

Spontaneity

All of this emphasis on planning doesn't have to rob you of your desire for spontaneity. Your lead time might be a little longer, but there are still fun things you can do on short notice.

One night when we were bored we got into the car and headed for Chastain Park, Atlanta's outdoor amphitheater. Willie Nelson was playing and the place was sold out, but we thought we might be able to hear some of the concert from outside the fence. Our going was so spur-of-the-moment that Michael was still in his mauve-striped pajamas and fluffy lambswool bedroom slippers (a tribute to how far he'd progressed from his long-pants-on-the-beach phase). I pulled up to the gate and finagled enough help to get him to a grassy hill where we had a lovely picnic in the dark, with Willie Nelson's voice filling the air around us. I worked at doing spontaneous things like that.

There are many trips you can take by car; many pieces of portable equipment fit nicely into the trunk or backseat. Some that are too heavy may require special attachments that can be rented or purchased. Michael had a battery-operated, three-wheeled vehicle (his "tricycle"), but I could not disassemble it and lift it into the car. When we discovered a secondhand hydraulic lift that attached to the car and held the tricycle, we were no longer bound to places where I could push a wheelchair. Mobility seems to generate freedom of thought. We could go to a trade show at the huge exhibition hall downtown, drive to a park with lovely gardens and long paths, or visit the children who lived nearby—without any advance planning.

If you want to be spontaneous in a larger way but have limited funds, it's worth checking into standby accommodations for flights and cruises. Many travel agents sell deeply discounted trips (50 or 75 percent off) one week before a planned excursion is to begin. Notify your agent of your interest and any special requirements, and wait for a surprise phone call.

Fun on a Shoestring

There are endless weeks and months when it is not practical or possible to engage in travel escapes. There are long, tough times for recuperation, rehabilitation, and hospital stays, not to mention financial constraints, but that doesn't mean you can't be creative and have fun.

The following things are free:

- Holding
- Massaging a back or a neck
- Drawings and notes from children and grand-children
- Reading aloud
- Playing board or card games
- Pushing a wheelchair
- A drive in the country
- Having a picnic—at home or in the hospital

Mike had three great pleasures: junk food, massages, and simply going out. The first two were easy enough to provide. The third took a little more energy, but he got such a boost from going anywhere at all that the effort was always worthwhile. When we went to New York for his son's wedding, he got enormous pleasure out of going up and down Fifth Avenue, just window-shopping. He also got a thrill from the hair-raising wheelchair rides his daughter gave him at the Plaza Hotel. The hallways were extremely wide and our room was a long way from the elevator, so she ran him down the hallway at breakneck speed. He loved it. Everything in his world went on in such slow motion that the sensation of speed and slight danger was wonderful.

We often go to great expense to explore the far reaches of the world while neglecting the attractions in our own backyards—those places we visit only when we have out-of-town guests. You can have wonderful day trips or half-day excursions that require minimal expense and only a short ride in the car. A simple way to expand your local horizons is to call the Chamber of Commerce and request brochures or pick up a local guidebook. Most states are looking for local business; mine even had a campaign called "Stay and See Georgia," targeted toward residents.

Holidays and Special Events

Just because someone is sick doesn't mean he or she has to miss out on the fun of holidays and family events—in fact sometimes he or she needs the involvement far more than the rest of us. But once again, some planning may be necessary.

When Michael's son was getting married in New York City, we had to find a hotel that could accommodate a wheelchair. Each of the five hotels we contacted assured us that it had accessible rooms but, knowing the low level of the general public's awareness, I asked our daughter-in-law-to-be to go to each one and ask to see a "handicapped" room. She immediately ruled out all but two of the hotels, and even the one we eventually selected had ten steps in front. The only way to get a wheelchair into the lobby was to use a side entrance that had only one step, go through a restaurant, and ride on two different elevators. That was the best of the selection! But the slightly complicated arrangements were well worth the pleasure Michael got from being able to attend the wedding.

Elaine's husband wasn't that fortunate; he was in the hospital when their son got married. Determined to include him anyway, Elaine called the telephone company to see what could be done. A special line linking the hospital room to the church enabled Roger to hear the service, and immediately after the ceremony he was able to speak with all of the guests.

A person who is ill or physically incapacitated shouldn't be treated with kid gloves. One year Michael's birthday fell just at the end of a hospital stay, and I knew people wanted to see him, so I planned a small party at home and invited family and close friends. One of the guests secretly arranged to have a belly dancer come over for a surprise birthday greeting. About an hour into the party, the doorbell chimes rang and in stormed the belly dancer . . . all three hundred pounds of her! Another time we had a New Year's Eve party—in February. Mike had been too sick to have our normal bash on the proper day, so we held the event a month later, complete with champagne and all the trimmings.

Much of the enjoyment of a holiday, event, or trip is the anticipation of it, but with all of the excitement many patients get thrown an unexpected curve. Jesse is all too familiar with the problem:

> Holidays, like Christmas, are very difficult for my wife. She forgets she is handicapped and tends to overdo. Everybody wants to do more than the other person, everybody tends to step on everybody else, and everybody is trying to make this one better than the last. I think that is compounded with us, because subconsciously we wonder if we will all be here the next time. It's no wonder that three of Pam's four heart failures have followed Christmas.

Another couple found a way around this type of problem:

> We no longer make any advance plans for Thanksgiving or Christmas holidays. We found after the first few years that Cynthia got herself so worked up about the plans that she made herself sick. Now we tread very lightly when approaching a vacation that she's really looked forward to.

Equally important is the realization that the letdown

after an event may yield unexpected stress for the patient who had a wonderful experience. This happened to Vicki and Brad:

> We were together for two weeks, just the two of us, which he adored. He had my undivided attention every waking moment. When we came back, I had a 7:00 breakfast Monday morning, a 7:00 breakfast Tuesday morning, a dinner meeting Monday and Tuesday nights, and a meeting Wednesday night that made me a little late in getting home. He was furious—just furious! I said, "Brad, this is the real world. Remember, you have just been living in fantasyland. That is what we have worked so hard for all year, to get a shot at fantasyland a couple of times a year."

If you are prepared for your spouse's letdown, you can help ease the way through it. Perhaps the best way is to make immediate plans for the next getaway!

Mind Games for the Other Fifty Weeks

Vacations and holidays are relatively easy to plan. One of the biggest challenges in helping your spouse cope with a long illness is day-to-day stimulation. Instead of a bulging calendar and pressing career, there is now just a long road of empty time stretching ahead. Many people need help in keeping motivated and mentally alert during the endless weeks and months of confinement—the other fifty weeks of the year. Vicki, after much searching, encouraged her husband to zero in on something that interested him:

> He has developed a few hobbies that have helped him, such as building and flying model airplanes, but he mainly just shops for the equipment to build them. He has a wonderful workshop, and that keeps him busy.

Elaine's husband had a long recovery time after two cancer operations:

He was really caught up achieving on the golf course, and to take that away left him aimless; he would just sit in the house. Then he got interested in photography, and when we took him to the golf course to sit and watch, he began taking pictures of friends and scenes there. For his birthday I built him a darkroom, which turned out to be a burst of genius.

Both of these caregivers picked up on an emerging hobby and helped with the development of the interest. These kinds of activities are excellent for patients who are physically confined or restricted but whose hand coordination is unaffected. Both the workshop and the darkroom can be built for minimal expense in a spare room, basement, or garage.

A creative outlet provides a good emotional release. As one patient says:

> It's important to express your emotions some way. It's real, real helpful, whether it be through writing or drawing or painting or whatever happens to be your thing. You don't have to be brilliantly good at it; you just need an outlet for your emotions, which otherwise tend to vary between tremendous extremes.

Cynthia, another patient, agrees:

> I used to say that it preserved my sanity just to be able to sit and draw or sew, especially in the beginning when I could get out of bed and do sedentary things for a few hours every day. My sewing was my outlet. I sewed for myself, for my friends, for my mother. I started sewing for a child whose parents were killed in an automobile accident so her foster parents didn't have to provide clothing for her. That was a big outlet for me.

The world of electronics and communications plays a significant role in mental activities for patients. Just look at what's available today:

Radio. My Aunt Mary was a baseball fan all of her life. Confined to bed when she got older, she often fell asleep listening to her team win or lose. For anyone with impaired vision, the radio can be a tireless companion.

Television. Since the advent of the television remote control unit, bedridden or wheelchair-bound individuals have great independence in switching through dozens of network and cable stations. Michael loved animal and underwater shows. He could escape into a TV world of travel and mobility and learn something at the same time. Rob, whose radiation caused such severe pain in his throat that he couldn't eat for weeks, became fascinated by cooking programs.

VCR. Over 53 percent of American households now have videocassette recorders, and the opportunities these provide are expanding at an unbelievable rate. For example, two hundred hours of classic television programming is now being distributed to local libraries, thanks to an innovative project of the MacArthur Foundation. In addition to supporting creativity and structuring the project, the foundation will be spending nearly a million dollars to coordinate and promote it on public television and radio. Anyone with a library card can rent these PBS (Public Broadcasting Service) and BBC (British Broadcasting Corporation) shows. In a separate project, the Carnegie Foundation is donating VCRs to six hundred public libraries so that people who don't have them at home can still have an opportunity to watch.

Our VCR enabled Michael to work from bed. Since his job had involved program purchasing for the broadcast company he was with, he could still make himself useful by screening and analyzing new television shows.

Computer. Computer networks provide hours of entertainment for shut-ins who are willing and able to learn how to access them. Any local college or university can provide information on how to learn, and many computer retail stores also offer training. But don't be discouraged by the thought of transportation to and from a course; most software packages have user-friendly instruction books, making solo home learning easy. New and used equipment is much more affordable today, and the latest laptop computers can even be managed in bed.

Audio Tapes. Audio tape services are growing with exponential speed. Most larger shopping malls have specialty stores with display racks full of books on tape, languages on tape, how-to-learn-anything on tape. Motivation, religion, overcoming bad habits, relaxation techniques—the list is endless.

A talking book service, The Cassette Library of the Hundred Greatest Books, is available from American Express and can be ordered by calling (800) 528-8000. The Mind's Eye is another company that sells audio classics, plus the BBC Audio Collection and other treats. Call (800) 227-2020 and ask for a catalog. On the lighter side, Cati Productions in New York produces romance novels that are acted out on audio tapes called "kissetts." They can be ordered by phoning (800) 666-CATI.

Ham Radio. Irene found herself in an embarrassing predicament when her husband's stroke damage caused him to telephone the same people over and over. She finally found a communications tool that saved her from total exasperation—a ham radio. She got it free through an operator who runs a special network for the disabled. "He now has the whole world at his disposal," says Irene of her husband. "He can call five million people with the same story."

Moving On and Letting Go

As the ultimate optimist, there are few things I am not willing to tackle, especially if they present a challenge. Sometimes, though, it is time to move on.

Our beloved Cayman Island vacations finally became too difficult. After Mike lost his second leg, our beach house took on the proportions of an Everest. There were steps everywhere, and where there weren't steps there were long stretches of sand. It was time to let go and move on.

I had to learn to let go in other ways, too. During the last two years of his life Michael spent most of his time at home, "retired from life." During the endless days and weeks he never *did* anything, at least not anything I considered worthwhile. He had only two pastimes: he watched old movies on television, and he read escape novels.

I couldn't stand watching such a powerful mind go to waste when there were so many constructive things he could have been doing. He could have been writing. He had already coauthored one book on radio and television programming, and he could have been writing articles in that field. With more than forty years' experience behind him in the broadcast and film industries, he had a lot to offer, had he only wanted to share his knowledge. He could have taken up painting, a hobby that was of interest to him because he loved wildlife and anything to do with the ocean. He could have painted scenes that were important to him. He could have developed any number of passive hobbies that would have stimulated his mind and creativity. Any time I suggested one, he immediately agreed: "You're right. I really should." But he never did. In order to encourage the writing I got him a computer, a tiny laptop model that he could have used even in his wheelchair. He never turned it on.

My main motive in pushing him was the hope that if I got him wanting something, doing something that he could manage and that interested him, it might give him something to look forward to. My ulterior motive was to occupy him so that he would not be so possessive of the little bits of time I had, because even when I was at home there were many things to do—housework or cooking or business-connected work.

After hundreds of suggestions and a year of frustration,

my efforts to motivate him were still not helping; all they were doing was driving me crazy. One day I realized that *you cannot want for someone else.* I could not impose my values on him—I had to let go.

I'm not saying that you shouldn't try to stimulate someone, to help him or her find something of value—a hobby or occupation—to latch onto. I think it's important to make every effort to help the person you chose as your lifelong companion add meaning to a life that otherwise seems void of excitement and accomplishment. But if your efforts are spurned, you must learn to let go. If you don't, you will suffer the extra burden of trying to push someone down a road he or she doesn't want to travel.

There was another issue at work here, too—one that took me a long time to acknowledge. I was trying to get Michael to do what *I* would have done in the same situation. I was so worried that he was wasting his mind and talents that I was blinded to the unique ways he entertained himself. It took one of the kids to point out to me after Michael had died that he did plenty of things to keep himself entertained. When we began renovations on the house to make everything wheelchair-accessible, he managed to stretch them out for nearly a year just because he loved supervising the workmen. He continually created things for them to do so he could feel useful and have company. After we moved to the house on Lake Lanier, he began putting out food to attract the ducks. Michael fell in love with those ducks and spent hours feeding and watching them. He even named them all.

His third hobby was, as his daughter puts it, "finding new ways to get stuck." He was as adventurous as it was possible to be in a wheelchair or a motorized "tricycle." One time he tipped over down by the dock and had to lie there and wait until someone found him. In spite of being bruised he wasn't the least bit upset, and in fact he told the story with great relish to anyone who would listen.

The point is, he did far more than I ever acknowledged. If I'd understood that, I would have backed off a long time before I did. Instead, I wasted a huge amount of energy with all of those Why Don't Yous, trying to project all of my wishes onto him. It didn't help him any, but it hurt me tremendously. *In order to maintain your own mental balance, you must let go of all things that are beyond your control.*

The very nature of a long-term illness creates emotional and physical cycles that are extreme, hard to predict, and difficult to comprehend when you are well and your husband or wife is sick or disabled. But the human need for involvement, entertainment, and exploration does not stop because of illness or disability. There are hundreds of creative, inexpensive ways to fill the hours and countless things to do and places to go when you plan ahead and utilize the advice of experts. Some of the travel ideas I have offered are not right for a patient who is bedridden, but others are suggested as engrossing mental activities when mobility is not possible or affordable. During those times it is especially important to plant the seeds of hope for adventures yet to come.

Bear in Mind:

Substitute new dreams for those that are no longer possible.

Go straight to the top if that's what it takes to open doors or change company policy.

Be creative. Today's travel and exploration possibilities are limited only by our imaginations.

Use visualization as a technique for working out logistics ahead of time.

Realize that the excitement leading up to a holiday, event, or trip can throw patients an unexpected curve.

Help your spouse find new hobbies. One of the biggest challenges in helping your spouse cope with a long illness is day-to-day stimulation.

You cannot want for someone else.

8
Taking Care of Yourself

W hen Michael told me you were in Europe, and he was at home recuperating from the loss of a leg, I thought, 'What kind of a person is this?' I didn't like you."

When an acquaintance expressed her honest feelings about my leaving Michael to go on a trade mission to Europe, I was terribly hurt and resentful. How could I have explained to her, or to anyone else, that taking care of myself and continuing with my life was necessary for my very survival? That my work was vitally important in maintaining my balance so that I could remain an effective, sensitive human being?

The pressure imposed by society is just one of the many important issues that must be understood and accepted before you can create a balanced life for yourself. I realize that my own methods of survival may seem selfish to some. I am not suggesting they will work for everyone, but I am confident that creative ideas and a positive outlook can make you feel good about taking care of yourself.

Looking Out for Number One

Caregivers often assume so much responsibility that they cease having a life of their own. They lose sight of the fact that if they are not on top of things and happy about who

131

they are, they can't care for someone else with any degree of competency. Years of intense, nonstop caregiving went by before Irene realized it would not be a crime to give herself a break:

> I finally feel that I can give myself permission to go and be with my mother on Christmas. She needs me, too. But it's taken five years to be able to do that, and I've been close to having a nervous breakdown most of that time.

Think how much easier those five years might have been had Irene learned in the beginning to look out for number one.

Frances is another caregiver who was imprisoned by her situation, although her confinement was not self-imposed. Her husband had Alzheimer's years before help was available:

> It sometimes got to the point where I felt I could not go on anymore. I would go into my backyard and actually scream at God: "If this is the kind of life you gave me, then please take it! I don't want it! I can't cope!"

Frances pushed herself until her own health was jeopardized. Her doctor finally intervened. "I have patients who are hospitalized with lower blood pressure than yours," he told her. "You might have a stroke going home. You've got to do something. It's either you or him."

Caring for a person with chronic illness is a stressful, long-term commitment. You cannot put every ounce of your energy, day after day, into the care of another person. Because you don't know how long your caregiving will go on and how much stamina will be needed over the long haul, you have to pace yourself. You must learn to conserve energy for important activities and to use outside help from the start so that you do not wear yourself out. Temporary relief and emotional outlets are essential, yet caregivers are often reluctant to do anything for themselves.

Vanessa, through necessity, realized the importance of help early on in her caregiving because she had not only an incapacitated husband but also a new baby to care for:

> One thing I would advise anyone else is to try to get as much help as you can. Either pay for it or line up your friends. There were times when I felt as if I was choreographing a long play that was my life: "You come on stage now, and you exit." I really did wind up utilizing and managing the people in my life to help me get through the day, get through the week.

Dr. Kitty Stein tries to get the ill person to take part in looking out for the caregiver:

> The sick person often feels that they're the only one in need. If they learn of other needs, they might be able to help in the problem-solving effort, to get the other person's needs taken care of. Even the therapist can be a collaborator with the ill person: "You and I have to figure out a way to help this person get her hair done," or whatever it is that is needed.

An additional benefit to this approach is that once the patient becomes an ally, the problem of guilt is alleviated.

Increased Dependence

The increased dependence of your husband or wife is a factor that can play havoc with your taking care of yourself. It is expected that you and the person you married can depend on one another, but when illness increases that dependence to a degree you never envisioned when you took your marriage vows, it's hard to know where to draw the line.

Michael's growing dependence made me realize that survival demanded a certain degree of selfishness—but the ensuing guilt was something I couldn't handle on my own.

I sought advice from my friend Vicki, who'd had years of experience with her own chronically ill husband. I asked her if she ever wants to run away:

> Oh yes, at least once a week. I just tell Brad, "Forget it, I'm tired of dealing with you." Or I might say, "This is all I can handle. You think about our disagreement while I go bake a cake or something." I actually never baked a cake, because I didn't want to mess up the kitchen and have to clean it up again, but I'd go read a book or do something constructive.

I found Vicki's spirit and humor uplifting. More than anyone else, she helped me understand that my gut feelings of self-preservation were not outrageous. She pointed out that I needed to maintain my own personality:

> Don't give in unless that is your typical way of behaving. I think we need to treat people who are ill much like we treated them when they were well. I couldn't change just because he had changed. I felt all the time that I had to be more of myself rather than less.

Katy finds that being sick and dependent actually puts pressure on *her*. She tries to minimize her dependence on her husband by encouraging him to find a life of his own. He now spends significant portions of the year working in another state:

> Maybe Ray's being away for parts of life is helpful sometimes. Not that we don't love each other, but it gives him room to deny things. It also doesn't put so much pressure on me. I feel better that he's getting on with his life, because that's always been my biggest worry. When you're married to somebody for a long time, you become very dependent on one another. I feel that if he is functioning independently, everything won't be quite so painful for him.

Being needed is a comforting feeling, but compassion

can turn to anger and resentment if you begin to feel like a sacrificial lamb. When Michael became physically dependent, it was a strange feeling for me. My very nature is one of independence. The physical side of his dependence was not a burden to me, but he quietly slipped into a state of mental dependence as well. I reacted quite strongly to that. Sometimes I left the house just to go to my office for some quiet time. I was still reachable by telephone, though, and once in a while he would call me just to say hello, just to reach out and know I was there.

SELFishness

Society says that when your loved one is sick, you must take care of him or her. Even if you pay someone else to help, you still have feelings of obligation. Leaving a dependent, sick spouse alone at the hospital or at home can cause guilt in even the strongest personalities. You feel as if there were a billboard with flashing lights outside your house, screaming to the world: "Selfish wife leaves helpless husband to pursue her own interests."

As a caregiver, you have a special need to focus on yourself now and then. Those caregivers we spoke with who had outside interests, a strong support system of friends, and physical or creative outlets were those who were coping the best. Those who had sacrificed everything to the needs of their husbands or wives were living in a cocoon of despair. Perhaps one of the most important gems of wisdom I heard on this subject was from a therapist who said:

> It's critical to be connected with SELF—that's with capital SELFishness. The caregiver tries to stay tuned in to the wants and needs of the disabled person at the expense of staying tuned in to his or her own wants and needs. So long as a person is connected to his or her own insides, he or she can simply look inside and say, "Is what's going on with my financial affairs/my sex life/the food I'm eating/the children/

the in-laws OK with me today? What is it in me that feels NOT OK?"

Take an inventory of all of your satisfactions and dissatisfactions. Don't succumb to the ease of thinking, "Of course I know why I'm so unhappy; I have to take care of my sick spouse." That's not quite all there is to it. SELFishness means you must have a sense of yourself in order to know what you need. If you get *your* needs met, you won't get resentful of your partner.

"Sure, it's easy for you to say," you may be thinking, "but how do I step back and take a personal inventory? What exactly is the thought process, and how do I learn?"

Stepping Back

The way for me to deal with the trauma of Michael's chronic illness was to run away from time to time, to step back. It was important not only to get away when I was at my wit's end but also to plan ahead so that I had something positive to anticipate. My stepping back depended on the mood of the moment and the depth of the Poor Me feelings. Sometimes I had to go off for a few hours, sometimes for a day, a weekend, or longer. I simply had to have time away.

If you can't step back on your own, a little help may be in order in the form of a nudge from friends. Joyce's close friends helped her run away whenever the hopelessness of her situation overcame her:

> Sometimes when Rob was really sick, I could feel myself withdrawing. My friends picked up on it right away. They'd call me up and they'd say, "We're taking you out. We're going to lunch," or "We're going skiing."

For you, stepping back might be a hike through the woods or an afternoon's quiet fishing on a lake, watching the cork bob up and down. It might be a half day of golf, dinner with a friend, or a movie. *Decide what is possible for you and what you want to do for your alone time—and then make the time.*

Miranda, a caregiver with a young child, found that a complete separation was necessary for her to take inventory:

> If we were going to get back together it was going to be based on the merits of our relationship and our marriage, not on the fact that he was ill. I did not feel a sense of duty to him simply because of his illness. I felt a sense of duty because I had married him. That was the stuff I worked through during the separation. I decided that our relationship had to stand on its own ground.

Miranda and Arthur did reconnect, but not before she broke free of the pressures of family and society to understand her own self.

Feeling like I am in control is important to me. It's part of what I believe in and teach. For over a year, though, I virtually lost that feeling. The only way to recover it was to step back in a really dramatic way. I signed up with one of the Outward Bound schools for a white-water rafting expedition on the Colorado River in Utah, an excursion that headed my list of "things I never want to do." The thought of being physically out of control terrified me, but because I had already lost the upper hand in my personal life, I thought that a direct confrontation with one of my worst fears might be the fastest way out of the bottomless pit I was in. I thought that if I could conquer that fear of careening down roaring rapids, I might also recover my former toughness once I got back on home turf.

My instincts didn't let me down. During the five-day expedition I realized the extent of the damage to my own self-image. I saw how the last two years had eroded my own decision-making abilities. *I also understood the absolute necessity of backing away from my everyday world in order to regain perspective.* Along with the others on my raft team, I learned about decision making, delegation, building a support system, planning ahead, and making contingency plans. Each one of those skills related directly to regaining control of my own life. I came away with renewed emotional strength, self-image, and confidence.

I am not advocating that each of you sign up to take an outdoor survival trip, but when you are in deep need of some good old self-analysis and desperately seeking an inner voice to give you direction and perspective, make a commitment to step back in a big way, to do something off the beaten path, out of the ordinary. If at all possible, make it a physical challenge.

Where's the Party?

It is very easy to let your social life slide. "Social life?" you say. "What social life?" Entertainment, friends, working out, and other personal activities form the backbone of long-term caregiving survival, yet they are the activities we most often push aside when the going gets tough.

Your social life, which should be the last thing to go, is unfortunately the first. From the day we met, Michael and I were quite different in our social needs. Once he came home from the office he did not care to be around other people, preferring only my company. But friends had always been an important part of my life, and once Michael became sick my friends became increasingly necessary for my happiness. Dr. Stein explains why:

> The chronically ill person needs friends, but the person who is the caretaker also needs a support system, sometimes very separate from the patient's. There's a need to talk about the reality beyond what your spouse's friends can deal with, without feeling pulled.

In addition to the comfort of close friends, you also need occasional social encounters. Bonnie, a caregiver whose husband had cancer, allowed herself to become reclusive:

> I tended to avoid social activities where everyone else
> was a couple. The idea of getting out is supposed to
> be an uplifting experience, but I found those times
> just reminded me sadly that I was a single spouse.

Joyce, whose husband also had cancer, experienced the
same initial discomfort but forced herself to go beyond it.
"When there were parties, I went by myself," she said. "At
first it was hard, but I got so that I could enjoy it."

Miranda found a way to get out without directly confronting the couples' scene:

> I love going to the ballet and symphony. At one point
> I wouldn't have thought of going to a Saturday mati-
> nee and leaving Arthur at home, but now I do it all
> the time. It lets me get out, so I don't resent the fact
> that Arthur doesn't like that sort of event. That's
> normal in a marriage; it has nothing to do with his
> illness. I am a much happier person because I do these
> things for myself without resentment. I knew myself
> well enough that I couldn't do it any other way.

I realize how limited spare time is, but an outside interest
may be the necessary catalyst to help you refocus. There
are countless ways to get out that don't require long-term
commitments. Pick *one* that interests you, such as a civic,
church, or synagogue activity, an industry function, a
garden club, the PTA, or a bridge group. Go on a good old-
fashioned shopping spree with a friend; if money is not
available for such an occasion, do what my family used to
do when we went to New York—window-shop at night
when the stores are closed.

Joyce carried on with her community projects, knowing
the diversion was good for her even though she sometimes
had to force herself to go:

> There were times I didn't feel like going, not because I
> didn't want to get out and go, but because I got tired

of all the questions I had to answer. A lot of times people asked and a lot of times they didn't, but I always felt they were going to ask. When they did— "How's he doing?"—I didn't want to reply with a casual answer, "He's just horrible." That wasn't the answer I wanted to give, even though that was true. It just wasn't my nature to make it nasty and gory to the general public. But I continued to support him and still got out a lot.

Creative pursuits offer another healthy outlet. Frances, whose husband had Alzheimer's before respite care was available, found herself confined to the house:

> It's a good thing I didn't turn out to be an alcoholic. That would have been the easiest way out, to drown my sorrows. Instead, I kept my sense by doing things, by keeping as busy as I could baking, cooking, arranging flowers in the garden, working with sea shells. I would try to be creative and make something beautiful, because I felt my life was so ugly.

Jesse, an executive, has an old barn that he is rebuilding:

> Hammering and digging, working on this project is one way I recharge myself. I also planted a small garden. It is such a welcome change from the office and provides physical activity with creativity.

Some caregivers have projects like Jesse's; others prefer to stay at home while a friend or relative takes the patient for an outing. Just being able to be home alone, to listen to music or read, is often relief enough.

Staying Fit

For me, one of the biggest challenges in taking care of myself was finding the time to keep fit. Physical fitness should be of concern to all of us, but the highly stressed life led by caregivers makes it crucial. Physical fitness leads to mental fitness. Exercise burns off all those negative emotions and leaves you feeling calm and yet alert, relaxed but energetic. Americans are obsessed with fitness, yet we tend to talk more about it than act upon our beliefs. And while it is hard enough under normal circumstances to find time to exercise, the time constraint seems prohibitive when you have a dependent spouse. Contributing to your apathy is a declining self-image. Why put any effort into looking good when the physical part of your marriage is waning or gone?

It was on my goal list: lose ten pounds. No big deal, right? Most people I know want to lose ten pounds. Then why had it been on my list for over three years? The logic and rationale are otherwise known as excuses: (1) Working out takes at least two hours (including getting there and changing clothes), and I really need to get home to be with Michael. (2) I worked longer at the office than I promised. I'd better zip home and fix dinner. (3) I'll ride my exercycle when I get home instead of taking the time to go to aerobics class. (4) I'll get up early in the morning for sure and ride the bike. (5) I'll go to the noon exercise class today instead of eating lunch. (6) I left my exercise clothes at home. (7) It's raining. (8) It's too hot. (9) It's too cold. (10) I'll be traveling for three days, and I will definitely use the workout room at the hotel. (11) It's been a rough week, I'm pooped. Poor Me, I deserve a rest.

Then Michele came to stay. She lived with us for a year to help out with her father while working on her master's degree, and she went to aerobics several days a week. Sometimes, for variety, she went to the three-mile path at the river to jog. Michele made me go with her all the time. Once in a while, when she was out of town, I'd even go alone! I got into good shape and was quite proud of my smaller dress size. Even though Michael was in the midst of surgeries and recoveries, with someone in the family to *make* me take care of myself, the guilt about investing time in fitness was gone. Through Michele *I discovered the neces-*

sity of having another person who shares your goal and helps you over the long haul.

Make yourself a thirty-day fitness goal; say, lose five pounds and get into better shape. Then find a buddy to commit to this with you—perhaps someone you've wanted to spend more time with anyway. Make a verbal commitment, or a bet, or set up a system of punishments and rewards.

Having It All

Now all you have to do is find the time to fit your workout into your schedule. Walk yourself through an average day: OK, I'm getting up out of bed, and Michael is still sleeping. What I'd really like to do is go jog, but I know that he will wake up in a little while and be hungry, and I'll need to get his breakfast fixed because he can't do it for himself. Damn the conflict! I want to do something for me. I want to go walk. Do I do it for him, or do I do it for me? Or—and this is where your ingenuity must come into play—how can I do both?

My solution to the dilemma was to put within Michael's reach everything that he might possibly need: a jug of ice water, some mouthwash, coffee in a cup on a cup warmer (or in a thermos), a piece of fruit, a bowl of cereal. A few feet away was a tiny icebox with milk and juices. He had everything he might need for the next forty-five minutes in case he awoke before I returned from my exercise. Then I went out and walked. *It is possible to take care of your spouse and to take care of yourself too. You can have it all.*

Still no time? It has long been doctrine that you have to exercise twenty to sixty minutes a day, three to five times a week, to reap benefits, but I recently read an article in *American Health* showing that even a short walk begins to reduce anxiety and blood pressure the very first day. You can get fitter by doing just twelve minutes of race-walking or other aerobic exercise three times a week. No matter how tight your schedule, don't you think you can find thirty-six minutes a week to do something nice for yourself?

Give Yourself Permission to Shut Out the Sadness

I have discovered in my seminar work with thousands of men and women that we are a society of permission seekers. We are overly polite and reluctant to make decisions without first asking someone else, "What do you think?" Whether we are ordering a meal at a restaurant ("Are you going to have a cocktail first?") or deciding what we need to take care of ourselves, we tend to rely on other people's advice whether or not those individuals understand our particular needs.

We need to reevaluate how often we ask permission and why we ask for it. When Michael was in the hospital he was sometimes angry and hostile. To stay there with him was unpleasant. It threatened to undermine the love and respect I had for him, so *once I knew he was being cared for by the hospital staff, I gave myself permission to leave.*

Elaine, whose husband had been ill a long time with cancer, used the same tactic when faced with an additional burden:

> My newly divorced daughter arrived on my doorstep. After a few days, I asked her to leave. "You're going to have to take care of yourself," I told her. "I'm very sorry, but I cannot take care of you right now. I'm trying to survive myself." I felt like a witch, but I couldn't bear the thought of sacrificing what was left of my life for yet another needy person. My pushing her away was necessary to my own survival. And rather than causing permanent damage, a better, more adult relationship developed as a result.

Give yourself permission to follow your gut instincts in order to get your needs met. Give yourself permission to reject situations that are depressing and self-destructive, if you have a choice. Learn how to compartmentalize your mind, to close one door that hurts and open another to continue living your life.

There are times in the roller-coaster cycles of long-term illness when it is unquestionably difficult to take care of yourself, but crisis times are not what we are focusing on; getting back to a degree of sanity is the issue here. When a crisis has subsided, it is time to create space and emotional outlets for yourself and learn how to do so without guilt.

There are many ways to ensure your survival and many little ways to reward yourself. Take a long, hot bubble bath with candlelight and music. Take a half day off. Play a round of golf. Play cards with your buddies. Go to a movie. Treat yourself to a massage or manicure. Use a multitude of treats to stroke yourself, to get your needs met. As soon as you have savored the moment of one, plan another for a few weeks away. Looking forward to these moments of pleasure is part of the process of survival.

The Alzheimer's Foundation has published a "Caregivers Bill of Rights." With their permission, I'd like to quote from it:

> We mandate the following rights:
> The right to live our own life to retain our dignity and sense of self;
> The right to be free of guilt, anguish and doubt, knowing that the decisions we make are appropriate for our own well-being and that of our loved one;
> And the right to love ourselves enough to have the confidence to do the best that we are able.

Looking out for number one should be a priority in your life. If you don't do it, who will?

BEAR IN MIND:

Look out for yourself. Caregivers often assume so much responsibility that they cease having a life of their own.

Let your spouse know you have needs, too. The sick person often feels that he or she is the only one in need.

Know where to draw the line. Illness can increase dependence to a degree you never envisioned when you took your marriage vows.

Don't be afraid to make time to be alone. You may simply have to have time away in order to regain perspective.

Maintain outside interests. Your social life, which should be the last thing to go, is unfortunately the first.

Stay fit even though you may feel there is no reason to put any effort into looking good when the physical part of your marriage is waning or gone.

Once you know your spouse is being cared for by the hospital staff, give yourself permission to leave.

9
Handling Change

When your life partner is chronically ill, your shared life changes forever. That's a simple statement but a profound, all-encompassing one. The more I lived with Michael—the more I saw, felt, cried over, and coped with all the havoc the diabetes was causing—the more I realized that our lives would never be the same as they once had been.

As Michael's illness persisted for months . . . and the months stretched into years . . . I began to learn what to expect. I noticed that in the midst of this chronic, forever-with-us condition there were definite ups and downs. Stages. Steps forward, and steps back. These ever-evolving changes in Michael's medical health, in our life-style, in our marriage—and in my own emotional stability—were part and parcel of the definition of chronic illness.

When I talked with other caregivers about the profound changes in their lives, I discovered that all of us faced common problems. Some of us, however, handled the waves of change—the chronic nature of our situation— better than others. And most of us handled things better some days than we did the next.

What made the difference? What made Rose, wife of a stroke victim, withdraw from her situation behind wry jokes and alcohol? What prompted Miranda to leave her husband, reconcile herself to his terminal illness, and return? What made Ann and Frank draw closer together, clasp hands, and face their very worst fears? And what made me, the eternal optimist and always the entrepreneur, push myself harder and harder until I found a turning point—very nearly a breaking point—where I knew a very important new business venture had to come to a halt because my energy was too scattered to carry it any further?

As I got to know other caregivers, I saw that some of us decided to let the changes brought on by our mate's illness sweep over us like a wild, destructive tidal wave. Others turned around, faced the waves of change head-on, and tried to ride them to the shore. Still others tried to deny the immense power of change—sort of like trying to build a seawall against the ocean's force.

I learned that we get bruised and battered, whatever path we choose. We cannot stop the waves, and we cannot alter their course. We cannot make our loved one's illness go away. *All we can control is our own response.*

Suddenly, all those old sayings I'd heard since I was three began to take on very definite meaning: Swim or sink. Bend or break. Adapt or die.

The Initial Blow

The most dramatic changes, of course, are in the patient's health. Over the course of three years my husband changed from a dynamic, robust man who loved to accompany me on long walks on the beach to a frail, mortally ill, double amputee. On the road from those beachfront walks to Michael's final months, I traveled without signposts, without a road map; nothing in my previous experience had prepared me for a meandering, stop-and-go journey through a life I naively thought was still my own.

Consider: When an illness first strikes and your spouse is at the critical-care stage, you hardly have time, much less the presence of mind, to think clearly about the future. By the time he or she has recovered enough to leave the hospital, everybody just wants to get back to the comfortable, familiar routines of home. But like thousands of other caregivers in similar situations, I quickly discovered that the familiar routines of home don't always work.

Caregiver Joyce, for example, faced an unusual dilemma that threw the entire household, including the family dog, out of kilter. Her husband, while recovering from the removal of a malignant sinus tumor, suffered from an unexpectedly severe and incapacitating postoperative headache. "He could not tolerate a normal voice—it was too loud for him," remembers Joyce. "If the dog barked, it sent him through the roof." To cope, she and the children spent most of their time away from the house or on the lower floor, trying to be quiet; even the poodle was banished to a cage outdoors. "This was the most stressful time of all," she says. "We had gotten through the surgery by knowing things were going to get better, but he was worse than he had been, with no explanation for it."

Riding an Emotional Roller Coaster

For the first few weeks after Michael lost his leg, I naively thought the crisis was over and things would eventually return to normal. It wasn't until he began trying to walk again, putting weight on his *other* leg, that we realized there were serious circulation problems with it, too. He was in constant pain. I tried to maintain a calm facade, but underneath I feared for the next stage—and the accompanying losses—which now seemed imminent. I had a great desire to run away from it all. What if, after this drastic, awful treatment, Michael continued to get worse?

As hard as it seems, most of us have to face the possibility that the illness *will* get worse. In this high-tech, quick-fix society, it's easy to focus on "miracle drugs" and heroic surgical interventions. We are programmed by television to believe in them. In the early stages of a disease, we become intensely dependent on what one cancer patient calls the "big guns" of state-of-the-art medical treatment.

But the return to so-called normal life at home without the buffers of medical technology can be more frightening than life in the waiting room of the intensive care unit. As Frank's wife Ann observes:

> At first you look forward to the end of treatment. You think, "If he can just get off this chemotherapy, we'll feel so much better." But as you get closer to the end of treatment, it's almost as if that's what you're holding on to. What's out there is a big, black space. As horrible as some of their side effects might be, the drugs and radiation are your friends—because once they're done, there's nothing between you and the cancer.

Frank endured an extraordinary course of medical treatment that began with a misdiagnosis of a type of lymphoma that would require a complicated surgical procedure during which he had "a 25 to 35 percent chance of dying on the operating table." Then he was told that he had non-Hodgkin's lymphoma and didn't need surgery after all. Instead, his doctors put him on extensive chemotherapy for six months, then recommended another four months of chemo and two additional courses of boosted radiation—and finally, a bone marrow transplant. Talk about emotional ups and downs!

After the transplant, which required eight weeks of isolation to prevent infection, Ann says that Frank was afraid to leave the safety of the isolation room:

> I had a hard time getting him to go out of the room. I got him into the anteroom, and he just stopped. I had to push, push a little more to get him to go out into the hall. He didn't like it at all out there. It was scary. He took about three steps and then turned around and went back in. We tried again later in the after-

noon and worked through that, but we were going from this one tiny, known environment to the huge unknown.

Like Ann and Frank, most couples go through a series of emotional reactions along with the physical changes: fear, depression, resentment, relief, resignation. "You go through a complete evolution," said one. For those dealing with an illness that periodically causes a crisis, this evolution can happen over and over. Katy is only one of many chronically ill people who routinely ends up in intensive care, fighting for her life:

> It's very difficult for most people to keep their marriage together. You just get some kind of balance, and things are going on nice and evenly, and then *crash*, you're back in the hospital. Each time I come home again the adjustments are tremendous.

If the marriage was rocky to begin with, the additional strain of constant change can tip the scale toward dissolution. Trapped in an unhappy marriage, Simon said that he felt sorry for his dying wife and tried to treat her kindly, but it wasn't always easy:

> You get where you resent it. You get very callous. A lot of times she'd have a seizure and she'd be there groaning and moaning, and I knew what was going to happen: she'd go through it, then start sleeping, and she'd wake up the next day and be goofy. When she was going through the initial two or three minutes of a seizure, I'd still be sitting there reading *Time* magazine. I was no longer terrified because I knew exactly what was going to happen. I knew it was going to happen until one day she died.

In some ways, Simon's blunt, honest expression of his feelings kept him sane. He didn't fall into the caregiver trap of denying his natural feelings while trying to be a saint!

In fact, *those who seem to cope best are those who can admit their feelings.* Knowing exactly where you stand emotionally can be the catalyst that helps you move on to the next stage. Fears and disappointments can seem less destructive, more familiar and manageable, when you know they're only part of a continuum and not a permanent state.

Claudia, who has multiple sclerosis, alludes to the sustaining power that this knowledge can give whenever her condition worsens: "When I let myself get a handle on it, know more about what's going on, I know that I've been in this place before. It's not news to me. The newness is gone." The depression Claudia experiences with each new setback has become a manageable, expected part of the disease: "When this started in 1975, the depression from an exacerbation might last three months. Now it lasts a week at most."

She has also chosen a different word to describe the feeling. " 'Depression' is probably not the best word for it," she says. "The right term is 'profound sadness.' " I find Claudia's word change very significant. "Depression" is sometimes viewed as a personal weakness, the last resort of someone who just can't cope. "Profound sadness," on the other hand, is a better, truer expression of an absolutely appropriate emotional reaction. The phrase implies a certain objectivity in understanding the situation, along with an acceptance of its emotional consequences.

Facing the Changes

As Michael grew sicker, our whole social/work/family structure—our vigorous, energetic way of embracing the world—seemed to be slipping from my grasp. I could hardly remember the sort of casual, spontaneous entertaining or spur-of-the-moment traveling we used to enjoy.

Painful as it was, I somehow had to accommodate Michael's chronic illness as a part of our lives, accept that it was here to stay, and learn to build a new and meaningful life for the two of us around it.

Rearranging the furniture of your entire life, I discovered, is not an easy task. But it can certainly be done—with help from friends, neighbors, hired household workers, employers, children, and even the patient.

"You get used to it very quickly," says Miranda, referring to the oxygen tanks and tubes that sustain her husband. Even their young son learned to crawl over and around the oxygen paraphernalia that runs through the house. This family's adaptive, "no big deal" attitude obviously helps them work around the illness in their daily lives.

Of course, each caregiver's individual circumstances are different. My own situation was symbolized by Michael's wheelchair. Among the challenges the rest of you may face are a spouse who is completely bedridden and dependent; a spouse who is ambulatory, but subject to crippling fatigue, pain, or other physical problems during any prolonged activity; a spouse who is physically active but suffering from a mentally devastating disease such as Alzheimer's; a spouse who often seems almost normal but several times a year faces a life-threatening crisis.

Vanessa's husband has stroke damage that interferes with many aspects of their lives:

> Until I learned what Dennis's limits were, even a simple trip to a shopping mall could be a disaster. At first, after he had been home a few months, I went merrily along, dragging him with me to the movies, a crowded restaurant, an outdoor festival. He wanted to get out, but once there, he was miserable—and too proud to say so. He was cross, anxious, impatient. And he kept disappearing to find the nearest bathroom—a habit that I knew was medically necessary (he has a neurogenic bladder), but that I sometimes found colossally irritating and embarrassing.

Vanessa's solution, which she stresses is still a "constantly changing experiment," is a compromise: shorter outings, frequent stops for food and rest, aisle seats in any public auditorium, and grocery shopping and other errands only at stores that provide public bathrooms. In short, she has learned to let Dennis set the pace. "If he slows me down—well, maybe I needed to slow down anyway," she says.

Often the patients themselves are the best judge of when old habits must change. This is demonstrated by Claudia's philosophical approach to the stages she faces in her battle with multiple sclerosis:

> I've chosen to call my recent car accident a milestone in the course of this disease. It's similar to the day I decided I needed to use the cane permanently: that required a personal shift from seeing myself as independently ambulatory to seeing myself as dependently ambulatory. The result is that I now have hand controls on my car.

If your patient is at all able to make decisions for himself or herself, my advice is to encourage this independence. In business, we call this style of management *delegating*. The great thing about delegating certain decisions is that you, the caregiver, stand to gain a little bit more free time!

Striving to Accept the Changes

Along with health and lifestyle changes, I had to continue coping with the changes in our marriage. With every new crisis that crashed over us and then receded, I felt our marriage changing its shape. Despite our best efforts, this illness was undermining the deep and satisfying marital balance we had achieved over years of living and loving together. Our relationship was altering itself daily in many large and small ways.

My independent, strong-minded Michael, homebound

and wheelchair-bound, was now almost totally dependent on me. He looked to me for everything from a glass of water to lively office gossip. He tried not to be too demanding, but his constant, unspoken need for companionship, for compassionate adult comfort in a time of great personal upheaval, was almost more than I could bear. My marriage, once a blessed source of strength, seemed in danger of sinking like a stone under the weight of Michael's illness. I looked around and realized that I had better start swimming or my love for him might sink in a sea of pity and resentment.

I have since discovered that many—perhaps most—caregivers entertain the notion of leaving. Miranda is one who actually *did* leave, for a time:

> I think there's a part of me that did not want to be married to someone who was going to die before me. I was blaming a lot of other, incidental things for our problems while unconsciously I was wondering why I should continue a marriage with someone I was going to lose. Why did I want to deepen the relationship if the person wasn't going to be here twenty years for me?

Miranda and Arthur separated for some time, and when Miranda left she took their new baby as well. After several months on her own she came to a more peaceful reconciliation with Arthur's situation:

> I think I grew up a little bit. I said to myself, Why would I rob this child of one moment with his father? We don't live in a perfect world, but let me make it as perfect as I can for as long as I can—meaning, let's be a family for as long as we can be.

If there's one lesson to be learned from this family's experiences, it's that different people express their true feelings in different ways. Katy, an asthma patient, says that her husband often can't face visiting her when the going gets really rough:

> Sometimes when I'm in the hospital Ray won't come and see me. He wants to run away. If you've ever seen somebody who is very close to you suffer—some people can deal with that, some people can't. If you love somebody, you feel so helpless because there's nothing you can do. Ray can't understand that just holding my hand, just being there, is being constructively helpful.

She is disappointed by Ray's running away but views it not as a sign that he doesn't love her, but as a strong sign that he does.

Of course, many caregivers themselves feel deserted—if not physically, then intellectually and emotionally. What hurt Vanessa the most was the crushing realization that she would never again be able to view Dennis as what he had been before the illness—her mentor:

> His work and mine were the same—we were both writers. But all of a sudden I couldn't count on his judgment. Whenever I asked his opinion of something I had written he would hand it back to me and say, "That sounds just fine." It was very frustrating. It was like the one person I needed in times of stress just wasn't there any more.

For a long time Vanessa was perplexed because Dennis didn't seem distressed by the catastrophic thing that had happened to him:

> Every night for about the first year, we talked and talked about it. I felt like I just couldn't reach him. I would even tell him that, and he didn't respond. Then in the course of one of these interminable talks I said, "I just wish I could get the old Dennis back." He looked over at me with the saddest expression in his

eyes and said, "Vanessa, the old Dennis is gone. He's never coming back." For the first time we both cried together over this horrible situation.

Although the moment was heartrending, it made Vanessa realize for the first time that Dennis had been agonizing over his illness as much as she had. Rather than hiding from it, he too had reached the same rational, if profoundly sad, conclusion. From that point on they started trying to build a new relationship.

The Expanding Circle of Change

Although Michael's illness did not crush us financially, for many couples the long-term financial impact of serious illness is often the single most devastating change of all. If the stricken spouse is the primary breadwinner, often both his income and the caregiver's income may be drastically reduced while their expenses are greatly increased. Elsewhere in this book I have suggested a step-by-step review of all financial resources available to the caregiver. This analysis is critical—as critical to your well-being as good medical care is to your spouse. Financial ups and downs, too, seem to be part of the definition of caring for the chronically ill.

For me, the most profound change brought on by Michael's illness was the change in myself. Somewhere during the course of his illness I came to realize that I would never be the same. Although he was the sick one, I eventually understood that I, too, was going through a terrible ordeal that would forever alter how I felt about myself and about the world.

Did I become stronger? That's a question I cannot yet answer. I thought I was already strong.

Did I become more compassionate? Well, I had always seen myself as a caring, responsive human being.

Had I been living in a Pollyanna world? Maybe, to a degree.

Did I need to be put to this sort of test? No. I didn't. And I wouldn't wish it on anyone. But I survived, and I did my best, for Michael and for myself. Let me explain.

Through most of these changes there was a profound feeling of loss: loss of health, of companionship, of beauty, of pleasure, and of time. There were days when I thought I was losing not only my handsome, virile husband but my own life. *My* life, the life I had chosen for myself and nurtured for forty-eight full, never-to-be-relived years.

As Michael's diabetes progressed, I sometimes felt that I was his only buffer, that I was the one who, by going through the routines of normal life, held this devastating illness at bay. Of necessity, I gradually assumed full responsibility for all household matters, for financial decisions, and for individual counseling with each of our six grown children. I also began taking on greater responsibility for my dear mother, who was clearly developing Alzheimer's disease. And against the odds, I tried to keep my business on track.

Finally, in the spring of my forty-eighth year—two years into Michael's illness—I snapped. I looked around me and saw for the first time that my business had to fold. That Michael was not getting well. That my mother was growing progressively worse. In despair and confusion, I ran away to our house at Grand Cayman and spent a week crying. Then, sitting in my torn chaise longue, watching the peaceful turquoise water wash over white sand and turtle grass, I reviewed the past two years and began to rebuild. The first step in the long process ahead of me was to admit that I had been suppressing my emotions for a long, long time.

I do not know whether all caregivers undergo so dramatic a change. I do know that the most successful ones, the ones who seem best able to balance caring for an ill spouse with sustaining a normal life, are the people with the strongest sense of self: self-preservation, self-love, self-reliance, self-confidence—on occasion even selfishness.

Not long after Michael's death, I was asked to give a speech before an audience of businesswomen. My topic was "Overcoming Roadblocks to Power," a subject I figured I certainly knew something about! One of the things I talked about was the relationship between change and power. Change can bestow power, I said, or it can take power away. Your own personal power depends a lot on how you perceive yourself and how others perceive you.

The changes in my life were disruptive and painful—and at times, more powerful than I was. But after a point, I could feel the tide changing. I knew then that I was strong enough to turn and face the waves.

BEAR IN MIND:

Be open. Those who seem to cope best are those who can admit their feelings.

Accept your spouse's chronic illness as a part of your life and learn to build a reasonably satisfying existence for the two of you around it.

10
The Importance of Attitude

W hen Michael lost the will to live, I planned a
party for him. During all the commotion of
putting it together, a dear friend of mine said, "You know,
Beverly, every time your world falls apart, you create
something from nothing. When you're handed a bunch of
lemons, you always manage to make lemonade." This
cliché typified a theme that I kept hearing over and over
again—that my attitude was very positive, very reinforc-
ing to Michael and to my friends and to all the people who
asked how we were doing.

Where do determination and strength come from? Those
who have a positive attitude will usually say that it comes
from within, that it is a part of their normal personalities
or philosophies of life. But I believe that it is something
you can learn and control.

Chronic illness can be a great destroyer of marriages.
Even if the marriage is strong to begin with, it is ever so
easy for one or both partners to develop an attitude that
eats away at the solid structure built up by years of hard
work. And if a marriage is foundering before illness
strikes, it takes superhuman effort to pull things back
together again.

A marriage can be strengthened by the commitment to
fight a medical battle. Many of the couples we talked to
spoke of rallying, and the people with positive attitudes

were the ones who coped the best. In spite of great adversity, they usually managed to find something positive in their life situations. If they were dealing with a serious illness, they knew someone with a worse one. If they attended support groups, they came away grateful that they were handling their problems so much better than the other people there. They tried to maintain as much normality as possible, refusing to let the illness dictate the entire structure of their lives.

Those who weren't coping were those who made little effort to get themselves out of their rut. They found numerous excuses to avoid outside help. They shunned support groups, counseling, and often even contact with friends, or if they did take advantage of these outside sources, it was often merely to unload. They had nothing positive to offer and were not receptive to ideas that might improve their lot. Cynthia, who has lupus, describes this tendency:

> I've seen so many people just wallow in self-pity. I get frustrated when I go to one of the support groups and listen to these people for an hour and a half. I think, "If you'll just stop complaining and try to do something, you might feel better." But they act like they're the only people in the world who've got lupus. I have a real short patience with people like that.

So do I. I have always been an "up" person, well aware of the effect of positive attitude on all life situations. Are you an "up" person or a "down" person? If you're the latter, I believe I can help you change your bad attitude into a good one. It won't be easy. It will take hard work, but there are any number of things you can do if you want to.

Ask for Help

Rose has been confined at home for the past nineteen years. You assume that she has a very serious illness, right?

But there is nothing wrong with Rose—it's her husband who has been disabled with a stroke. Rose has fallen into the role of martyr, of Poor Me. She has given up her job, her outside interests, and most of her friends, not to mention her freedom and her self-respect. She sits in a small apartment, year after year, caring for a man who verbally abuses her and whom she no longer loves. She has a chip on her shoulder the size of a California redwood tree. "I've been angry so long I'm worn out," she moans.

You can't help but feel sorry for Rose in her self-created helplessness. Self-created? Yes. Rose had a choice.

Help is available. All you have to do is reach for it; ask somebody to throw you a line. Do people call you, asking what they can do? Take them up on their offers! They feel helpless and sincerely want to lend a hand. Identify what needs to be done and delegate it. Try it just once; you have nothing to lose and plenty to gain.

Call a friend. At the very least you will have an ear to listen; at best you might be led to something or someone else. Your friends are tired of hearing your complaints? Try joining a support group made up of others who are experiencing a situation similar to yours. It's amazing how much relief comes simply from knowing that you aren't alone in your misery. Are you convinced that a support group will have nothing to offer you? How can you be so sure if you've never attended one? Don't you owe it to yourself to go *just once* before you form an opinion?

If you need a reality check on how well you're handling all the emotional stress in your life, consult a professional. This doesn't necessarily mean signing up for costly and lengthy therapy. It is possible to ask a psychiatrist or psychologist for an evaluation. My consultation with a psychiatrist reinforced my own belief that I was coping extraordinarily well, but if that had not been the case she could have recommended any number of options other than private treatment—group sessions, perhaps, that are less expensive than private treatment. See Chapter 15 for more detailed information on finding counseling.

Don't Get Sad—Get Mad!

Give yourself permission to feel a range of emotions, whatever they are, whatever you're feeling. Claudia suffers from multiple sclerosis:

> Once when I was telling my doctor how depressed I got, he said, "Don't get sad, get mad." That was very empowering to me. And anger is appropriate. The frustration is that there's nobody to be angry at. If people are God fearing, then they can be angry at God, but in general people aren't or don't think of it that way, so there's nobody to be angry at. Most people don't get angry—they just get sad.

But many people are afraid of anger, fear, resentment, and other "bad" emotions, afraid that if they give way to such intense feelings something terrible will occur. What they don't realize is that the mere expression of negative emotions helps to dissipate them and to open the way for other, more positive feelings to emerge.

For me, getting visibly upset is a big deal because I am not a confrontational person; my feelings are within. The one time during Michael's illness that I did lose control caused quite a scene. My son was over for dinner, and halfway through the meal the atmosphere at the table began to feel like a battle zone because of an issue between Michael and me that kept building and building. He was attacking me for something—working too hard, or whatever—and I finally got upset enough that I excused myself and left.

I grabbed a box of Kleenex, ran out on the deck, and broke down—just cried hysterically, on and on. After a time I realized that nobody knew how upset I was, and that made me even angrier. What good did it do to be upset by myself? I took my box of Kleenex and went storming through the kitchen, screaming something as I went, then jumped into my car—which happened to have the keys in it—and screeched out of the driveway.

The only problem was that I had left my purse behind. Now, there is absolutely nowhere you can run away to without any money. I could not even call a friend to see if I could come over and spend the night, because I didn't have a quarter. I didn't have a credit card; I didn't have a dollar. I only had my box of Kleenex. After an hour of driving around crying, I had to go home.

The point I'm trying to make with this embarrassing story is that here I was, all this time, thinking how in control I was and how well I was doing. Then, at the slightest nothing, I suddenly exploded. I made quite a fool of myself, but *I felt hugely better* a day or two later because all of that pent-up anger and resentment—which I hadn't realized existed—was out of my system.

It is easy for you to feel that you are going crazy. One day you want to do the world for your spouse; the next you want to throw him or her out of a ten-story building. It is a long haul, and your feelings can change. You've got to roll with the tide in order to survive. If you're vacillating all over the place and think you're going crazy, relax. Anger and frustration are natural reactions to the changes and stresses in your life.

Acknowledge your anger. Talk it out. If you can't unburden yourself to your friends, seek a professional. That's what they get paid for. Work off your resentment. Go stomp around the neighborhood for half an hour. Let it all out.

Be a Positive Person

Jesse raised four small children while his wife was suffering from a severe heart condition that could have killed her at any moment, yet he never let the thought of what might happen get him down:

We can control our attitudes more than most people

realize. I can control what I think. I've had my ups
and downs in both business and family relationships,
but I don't let that bring me down. I just pick myself
back up and say, "Hey, you gotta get going again."

I use a visualization method. When something goes
wrong, I always visualize that something will be
better from it. I never see my wife as being sick. I see
her as whole. I see her as bubbly and being full of
energy. And that carries over to her.

The wonderful psychiatrist in New York whom I talked
with from time to time uses visualization as a positive
therapy technique. I recall that once when Michael was at
home and totally dependent, she told me how to create my
own private space when I wanted to run away and couldn't:

> Go into a room alone, if possible, and close the door.
> You're closing out the rest of the world from *your*
> space. Now visualize a ring, a circle around you,
> almost like the planet Saturn. When you are inside
> that ring you are safe. You are alone. You are at peace.

Admittedly, when I first heard that, I chuckled quietly in
amusement. One sleepless night, as I lay in bed listening to
my husband gasping for breath, I decided to try her silly
idea. It not only worked in a room alone, it truly helped in a
middle-of-the-night, restless situation.

You do have choices. Your present and your future—more
simply stated, today and tomorrow—will be positive or
negative based on your own mind. Being a caregiver, you
often feel like you are trapped and you have no choices or
options.

From the bottom of my heart, believe me, you do have
options. The Bible says, "Know thyself. Whatsoever you
think of in your heart, you are." Napoleon Hill, noted
author, states, "Whatever you vividly imagine, ardently
desire, sincerely believe in, and enthusiastically act upon
will inevitably come to pass."

How Can You Become a Positive Person?

If all the lights look red, then you must *find an outside source* to help change them to green. Something as simple as a newspaper can be uplifting if you look for the positive stories. The sports section is good for that; it is full of heroes, people who have risen from ashes to stardom. Take strength from those personalities.

Read biographies. They are wonderful ways to remotivate yourself. If you're a listener rather than a reader, get books on tape, now widely available at bookstores or libraries. If the only spare time you have is during those trips to the doctor, listen to tapes in the car. When you need to be lifted, try motivational tapes.

Start a new hobby or activity that involves an emotional or mental commitment. Tackle something that stretches your imagination. Learn a language. If you'd like to expand your mind but can't get away from home because you're busy caretaking, take a correspondence course. It's inexpensive and you can fit it into your own schedule.

There are any number of ways to become a positive person. The aim is to *do something that will refocus your thought process outside yourself and your own problems.*

Vanessa uses a historical perspective to remain positive:

> In the great sweep of human history, there were so many people who had worse things happen and who lived on and accomplished things anyway. They were totally alone. There were no telephones out on the prairies in 1892. There was no nursing agency to call up, either, to come relieve you for a while. That has helped me maintain a perspective. Sure, life is hard, but it's only in the last forty or fifty years, with the advent of psychologists and of very secure, well-off Americans, that humankind has expected life to be rosy all the time.

Do It Now

Do everything today. Don't put it off. Don't wait until your spouse is better, it's not raining, or you can spend more money. Most of us spend our lives waiting. Look at each of those things you're waiting for and see whether you really need to be doing it right now, either by yourself or with your spouse. Take that vacation, learn Chinese cooking, start that perennial garden, learn about other cultures. Why wait?

When Arthur first found out that his time might be limited, he rushed to do some of the pleasurable things he had always been putting off—like buying cars and racing them and traveling:

> I wanted to do everything now, everything I knew I wouldn't be able to do in the future. Financially it may not have been a good idea, but I don't regret any of it. It's true that there are advantages to being ill. I've done an awful lot of things too many people put off until they're in their fifties or sixties and they've had a heart attack, and they suddenly realize it's too late. At least in the last ten years I've done those things.

Vicki and Brad also chose this route—a path they don't regret:

> We were leading a contemporary life, managing a home, a child, and two careers. It read like something out of *Vogue* in 1972. It was fun, exciting, and different from any other generation. Then all of a sudden, *Pow!* It was as if somebody said, "You guys have had enough fun. Come to grips with the real way of life."
> For a brief period of time there was a great deal of resentment: Why at age forty-seven? Why not sixty-seven? That is when we decided we would do the one thing we both had always wanted. We had always said, "We'll travel later." Suddenly realizing that there might not *be* a later, we decided to do it now. Three

years after Brad's first stroke we went to Europe. We have seen the world over the past twelve years during my vacation times from my job.

Do everything you want to do now and say everything you want to say now. Don't find yourself years down the line thinking, "If only I had said . . . " This doesn't apply only to saying, "I love you." You can also say, "I'm sorry you haven't been able to play golf for the past five years. I know how much you used to enjoy it." An expression like that is just as effective to let your husband or wife know how much you care.

Reassess Your Goals

You are probably aware of the effect that goals can have on the will to live. Unfinished business can become one of the major things keeping someone going. Louise has been treated for a brain tumor that is now in remission:

> My reason for living is to get my goldurned kids raised so that Jeffrey doesn't have to do that. He really is a good dad and a good helper, but he needs more than just himself. He can't do it on his own. I want to make sure that my children are all grown up. I want to be there to see it.

She probably will. I know of a "terminally ill" woman who kept going for eight years because she was determined to see her youngest daughter finish high school.

Goals are equally important for the caregiver; in fact, I'd say that *the single most important thing I can open your eyes to is the absolute necessity for setting personal goals and priorities relating to yourself and to your life together with your ill spouse.* If you do not have goals, you do not have anything to look forward to. Now, more than at any other time in your life, you need a reason to wake up each day. You also need to focus your attention on something other than the sick person you are caring for, *focus on something to look forward to.*

Most people think they have goals but don't. What are yours? Have you ever listed them? I have a page in my notebook that lists short-term (the next few months), medium-term (a year), and long-term (two to five years) goals. I make a point of referring to it once a month to assess my progress.

There are four criteria that I consider important when setting goals: they must be realistic, they must be attainable, they must be compatible with those of your spouse and family, and they must be measurable. I have eight categories on my goal sheet: mental, physical, spiritual, family, financial, career, social, and miscellaneous.

Just to give you an example, let's look at my list of short-term mental goals. I want to stimulate myself intellectually, but instead of saying, "Read more," I specify, "Read one book a month." I want to learn desktop publishing, which will require nothing more than a two-hour course plus some work at home. I want to organize my financial records, so I have set a deadline for getting that job done. And I want to learn to be a better time manager. These are current goals, but they all would have been attainable even while Michael was still alive.

When Michael became ill, none of my goals changed. But I obviously couldn't do everything I had planned, so how did I manage? *I learned to set realistic short-term goals for myself.* For example, I had a goal of accepting a speaking engagement in a foreign country. When Michael became critically ill, it became important for me to take it off the short-term goal sheet so that it wouldn't become a negative. I didn't forget it altogether; I simply moved it to my long-term goal list because I was aware of how much I might resent Michael if I felt he had affected something I so badly wanted.

Building my business was another important objective for me, but I could not do that for the twelve months stretching ahead of me so I took that one off my short-term and medium-term goal lists as well. Instead of thinking myself a failure each month when I looked over my goal list and saw I'd made no progress in this area, I just moved it a little further into the future. Let me assure you that making that move brought a lot of pain and disappointment, but by doing so I prevented it—as much as possible—from being a constant source of negative drain. It made all the difference in the world. *Eliminating the sources of negative drain whenever possible is just as important as creating the positive sources.* You must create goals that are reachable.

The importance of flexibility became a goal of its own. So did the idea of not setting long-range goals. I had to accept the thought that putting my career and achievement quest on hold for the next year was OK. Along with that went a conscious decision to give myself permission not to make any commitments, not to move forward. The year ahead was going to be totally contrary to the last twenty-eight in business, but that was a specific tool I used in order to keep from resenting what was happening. I put it all into a definite time frame: "I will do this for twelve months and then reassess."

None of my goals changed; they only moved to the other list, and I created other short-term goals to replace them: to lose ten pounds was one, to stop eating myself into oblivion, and to become a stronger, more fit person. I set a realistic schedule to do it: one visit a week to a fitness club and three walks a week, rain or shine (well, maybe not when it was raining). Michael would be fine during that time frame.

My short-term social-goal list became another way of building up my support system. "Have Faye and Bob for dinner one night this month," I wrote. Michael and I hadn't seen them lately; we wanted to be with them. Even if we had to order out for pizza, I was creating a time with friends rather than sitting back and saying, "I'm lonely. Poor me."

If your time is constrained, try combining two goals. If one goal is to get fit and another is to see a friend, invite the friend to join you on your walk or when you work out so that you can maximize your time.

One of the most important areas to attack if your spouse is chronically ill is *financial matters*. Itemize the things that you need to change or to get a handle on. Analyze what you need to do and then set up a plan to do it. This focuses on the reality of getting it done without making it a big deal: "I need to update my will. I need to get it done within three months." Make it a project.

Take One Day at a Time

Today is an important time. You must develop a frame of mind that encompasses that thought. Try to recognize that every day has, somewhere in it, a gem of a moment. Because I am such a goal-oriented person, this was something I had to make a conscious effort to learn. I began to keep a diary to help me focus on those moments. It might have been that Michael made his own lunch or that he took his first step or simply that he didn't regress that day.

The strong patients and caregivers we spoke with shared this one-day-at-a-time attitude. They focused on the positive events of each day rather than on the long-term, possibly bleak, future. Miranda's husband has been given two years to live:

> I think about it from time to time. I'm aware of it. But I don't dwell on it. If I do, then I'm going to spend the rest of his life having him die instead of enjoying living with him. I've really gotten into the good old day-to-day living and taking one day at a time—not taking it in an I-made-it-through-another-day way but just enjoying each day.
>
> There was a period of time when—and I don't think this was necessarily due to his illness, I think that all of us go through this in our lives—I focused so much on the future. What's going to happen? Am I going to be happy five years from now? How many

children am I going to have? That kind of thing. You can get so wrapped up with futures and worrying about futures that you don't do anything about today.

Stop and Smell the Roses

Loss of health requires a certain amount of grieving—for the spouse and family members as well as the patient—as does any loss, but it helps to keep the loss in perspective. Dr. Kitty Stein says:

> The one thing I offer people is the reminder of the difference between loss through death and loss through illness. When there's a death it's final— there's nothing else. When there's a loss through illness it feels a lot like a death, but the difference is that you still have something to hold. You've got to mourn what's lost, but you also need to understand what's still there.

In other words, there is always something positive to find in every situation. It helps to realize how much worse things could be. This gives many people the bright outlook they need to carry on. Arthur views his lung disease this way:

> I count my blessings from the standpoint of how lucky I am. There are an awful lot of things I have and can enjoy that other people will never have.
>
> I am uncomfortable sometimes that there are things I can't do. There are frustrations with dragging equipment around. But there was this girl I knew who died in October, and I know several other people who have nonoperable, terminal cancer. It puts my own illness in perspective. There are bad days when I don't really feel that I want to go anywhere, but it could be much, much worse. You start sounding like you're talking platitudes after a while,

but it is absolutely true. Most clichés have more than a little truth in them, and this is one of them: there's always somebody worse off.

His wife adds:

None of us has guarantees in life. Enjoy the good times while you have them. I said to Arthur the other day, "If we could freeze time, this wouldn't be a bad time to freeze, because everything is going so well with everybody." But it's times like this that help us get through when there's going to be another bad time.

Get Acquainted with Your Stroke Count

I need a certain number of positive strokes each day in order to feel good about myself. Let's say that on an ordinary day it takes a hundred positive strokes for me to end up on a positive note. If saying "hello" and getting a friendly "hello" back is going to give me five strokes, then I have to do a lot of greeting in order to get up to a hundred. If getting a hug gives me twenty strokes, then if I hug five people during the day I've fulfilled my quota. But if, when I come home, somebody sick is going to say, "I've had a terrible day. Where have you been?" then that's a negative fifty strokes, and I'll have to work a lot harder during the day to build up enough strokes to cancel that out.

You must become aware of what is going on in your own mind in order to fill that stroke count, to create a balance, and to move forward. You have to have a realization of what will make your count go above neutral. You know what's going to take it down—waking up or coming home to a very dependent person—but you have to learn what will build it up.

There are many ways to build your stroke count. One is picking up a phone and calling somebody—that might create fifteen positive strokes. Another is getting a compliment. And if getting a compliment makes you feel positive, then giving one first might yield something back. That is a way to create a more positive attitude.

If you're dragging, then your stroke count is low and you've got to figure out how to get what you need in order to get it back up again. You aren't going to get it from your dependent, chronically ill spouse. You have to figure out what you need and how often you have to have it and where you're going to get it.

Many of us do this every day without being aware of it. If you know that you need to exercise three times a week in order to feel good, that gardening or cooking or playing with the dog gives you a lift when you're down, you are already using this technique. You just have to use it a little more consciously when you're facing a constant emotional drain at home.

Giving is one of the best techniques for building up your stroke count. Ask yourself what you can give today. You might think, "I'm already giving all I have to this person at home; I can't possibly give any more." But *there is a difference between giving out of necessity and giving because you want to.* If you give of yourself, the appreciation of others makes you feel good. Do you think you don't need a support group? Then go to a meeting with the thought of giving rather than taking, of sharing rather than unloading. Share with others a trick you have learned to keep your family's spirits high or a unique way of dealing with anger and resentment or a recipe that even a sick person can't resist. If you get ten Thank You's and each one is worth fifteen points, you're coming back with far more than you gave, and you're stoked up for what you have to face when you get home.

Lighten Up!

We always called Michael's three-wheeled vehicle the "tricycle," and when he got his first prosthesis we called that his "training wheels." "Michael got his training wheels today," I would tell my friends and the children. "You ought to see him whip around the house!" It made other people feel more comfortable.

A good sense of humor is just one facet of an overall good attitude. If you can manage to keep yours, it will boost everyone's morale. It may even do more than that. According to one psychologist, "Laughter puts people into an altered state of consciousness where their body is open to healing psychologically as well as physically." Lighten up the situation whenever possible.

We discovered that one of the great benefits of being with somebody in a wheelchair is that you can go to the front of any line. When we went to Disney World we immediately went to the front of all those incredibly long lines, and whenever we returned from our house on Grand Cayman we were the first through customs. We joked about putting a sign on Michael—"Available for rental to go to the front of the line." We talked to him like that in order to lighten up the situation. We even called him "Rent-a-Mike."

If your spouse can't take quite that degree of humor, try more subtle touches. Michael was in the hospital for Halloween, and one of the kids brought in a little Snoopy dog wearing a mask. Instead of sticking it on the window ledge we hung it on the IV so that the nurses could comment on it.

Handicapped people often walk a thin line between annoyance and hilarity. Arthur finds that lapsing into absurdity can often diffuse a potentially tense situation:

> When I fly, I go in a wheelchair down to the gate. People tend to believe that someone who is in a wheelchair or someone who is physically handicapped is also mentally handicapped. I'll be with a friend of mine, and we're both dressed in business clothing, and people will say to my friend, "Does he want . . .? Would he like . . .?" as though I'm incapable of either speaking or thinking. I've had some fun with that. One time in the airport baggage claim, when a couple

of people had done that, I stood up and proclaimed loudly, "It was a miracle! The money I sent to Jim and Tammy Bakker paid off!" and walked out of the airport.

Cynthia and Ben use laughter to lighten the effect that her lupus has had on their marriage:

We've learned how to laugh at a lot of the situations and just make the most of them. I was always complaining about how fat and ugly the drugs had made me, because that's how I saw myself; I had been a small person all of my life. Ben would say, "That's OK; we'll just buy your gowns at Fashions for Fat Folks." He could have said, "Oh, honey, I'm going to love you no matter what size you are," but I didn't need coddling. I needed somebody to remind me that I was a happy person.

If you're still unable to find any humor in your own situation, get some humorous tapes, and listen to them with your spouse, and remember how much fun it is to laugh!

Use Your Beliefs

Until I was forty-five years old, I never had down periods. I was a true optimist, almost innocently blinded to the harsh realities of the world. Both parents were alive, and no close friends had ever died. When Michael became sick, I needed a source of strength outside myself.

When a life-threatening crisis strikes, most people either turn to religion or reject it. They rarely sit in the middle. How they deal with the ever-present Why Me? is usually the deciding factor.

For some, religion gives strength to cope with the crisis. Jack lost his wife to diabetes:

I don't know how to explain. I think that God just

gave me a lot of strength. It seemed that no matter
how bad it got, I just accepted it and could handle it
somehow. It was really hard and miserable, but no
matter how hard it got it seemed like I could take it.

I also fell into this category. I was born into a particular
religion but practiced it to a very limited degree until
Michael became sick. Then, like many others, I turned
slowly, quietly, and steadily to religion. Over the five-year
course of Michael's illness, I received strength from expressing what I was feeling to one particular friend and got
Scripture and verse in return. I listened to tapes and found
messages of comfort and peace in them, helping me to
build up a reserve. I began to realize how much strength I
could draw from spirituality. It helped me deeply and still
does.

Michael, too, turned from a great distance of nonbelief
to find strength in God. He didn't get nearly as far as he
might have, but for him it was a longer road. He at least
went far enough to find great strength, great comfort, and
peace about his past, his present, and—most important—
his future.

Some, like Arthur, aren't themselves believers but still
acknowledge the power of faith:

> I am not particularly religious. My wife is, and I think
> that's helped her a lot. That's something that's been of
> value to her. I don't share that right now and I would
> be hypocritical if I went to church every Sunday and
> professed great faith that I don't have, but it's helped
> her accept some things. I honestly wish I could feel
> that way.

At the other end of the spectrum are those who take a
medical and scientific approach to the Why Me? question.
Cynthia was a nurse before her illness:

> I hear so many people who think that God planned

things for them. I don't believe that I was bad in 1982 and that God punished me by deciding I was going to be diagnosed with lupus. I don't subscribe to that, nor do I believe that I was just waltzing along happily through life and was suddenly stricken with some illness. I have a belief in God, and yet I think that there is a scientific basis for what happens. What I do believe is that I was born with some kind of defect in my immune system, and because of exposure to either environmental factors or viruses that have come into existence in my generation, and things that I may have done—like exposing myself to certain chemicals—I think that all of those factors may have triggered enough of a response from my immune system that it set the lupus in motion.

Some people delve beyond religion and known science into psychology and the powers of the mind. Katy has been struggling with severe asthma for the past twenty-five years:

> I was taught self-hypnosis at a very early age to try and control my disease. I still firmly believe that if I hadn't combined both the mental therapy and the physical treatments, I wouldn't be here today.

Whatever your beliefs, now is the time to confront them, to analyze what they are, and to use them to your advantage. Whichever way you decide to turn, you may find the strength needed to add richness and staying power during this challenging period in your life.

Don't Be an Ostrich

All through Michael's illness I made a substantial effort to plan trips, both day trips and out-of-town trips, so we would have something to look forward to. We both got an incredible amount of strength from going to our house on Grand Cayman, so we went there as long as we could.

When that was no longer possible, I found a substitute. It was vital that Michael continue to do what was most meaningful to him.

Just before he lost his second leg, we actually went to Europe. He had been only once before, during the Second World War, so he had never "been to Europe" in his memory other than during that negative experience. I wanted him to be able to go, so we accepted an invitation to a conference in London.

It wasn't as though he was feeling fine. Pain was omnipresent in his "good" leg, so he was restricted to a wheelchair most of the time. It was not an easy trip to plan or negotiate. It would have been much easier to stay at home once it became awkward for him to get around, but I wanted him to have something to look forward to and to do things he had never done before.

Arthur sets another good example. He must breathe oxygen most of the day, and this involves carrying a tank around with him wherever he goes:

> There are a lot of people, especially older people, who, when they first have to start on oxygen, will never be seen in public. They never go out again. But I won't hide it or disguise it, and I will not avoid doing things. I like to go to good restaurants. I do some things where you will not often see people who are disabled or on oxygen, so it attracts a little attention that way. I almost flaunt it at times: "Yes, I'm on oxygen. What're you going to do about it?" It's probably healthy, to a point, because it says that I refuse to give in. I refuse *not* to be seen in public.
>
> I think if I ever get to the point where I don't want to go out or get ashamed to be seen or don't want to deal with it, I'll be in real trouble. That will be when I start to give up on things.

It is vital that you get your spouse—and yourself—out and about as much as possible. Don't let the logistics imprison you in your own home. If you want to get out, you can. Nothing is better for you both than the anticipation of an outing and the regeneration of spirit that it provides.

Educate Yourself

Knowledge is the key to control. The more you read, the more questions you ask, the more you listen, the more you watch television health shows and cable channels like Lifetime— the more you will be in control in emergency situations. You should be even more familiar with your spouse's condition than the doctors are. No one else spends as much time with the patient as you, and you have the benefit of consulting with *all* the doctors, something that they themselves often fail to do.

On several occasions when he was in the hospital, Michael became delirious and the doctors couldn't figure out why it happened. I was the only one who'd had enough continuity in his care to figure out that whenever they added codeine to the other pain medication they were giving him, it made him crazy. If I had not been there, aware of every detail of what was going on, I would not have discovered this. From then on I could tell them, "Under no circumstances give this man codeine." Because I knew what I was doing, I could take control.

Both you and your spouse must educate yourselves about the illness you are fighting. With many diseases, damage can actually be minimized by careful control. If early signs of impending problems are noticed, they can be swiftly dealt with before major organ systems are involved. Cynthia, the nurse with lupus, is well aware of this:

> It's important to learn as much about your illness as you can; then you learn to live with it a lot better. Some people don't even want to know what they've got. There's no way you can deal with an illness if you don't know what you're dealing with. I firmly believe

that if you're given the diagnosis of a chronic disease, you must learn all that you possibly can about it. Learn to live with it, rather than having it control your life.

Denial: A Hindrance or a Help?

Michael was a denial person. In spite of knowing since childhood that he was diabetic, he smoked, drank socially, ate badly, and shunned exercise. Denial—refusing to acknowledge an illness or the severity of an illness—is an issue that crops up again and again. Michael's denial made him a difficult patient to treat, especially when he continued with most of his bad habits while his diabetes slowly consumed him.

Denial can cause massive problems for the caregiver as well. Irene is married to a diabetic who refuses to admit that he is sick even though he has lost both legs to the disease:

> He doesn't want anybody to think or say that he's an invalid. It took nine months for him to let me put the handicapped sticker in the car window. I would have to push the wheelchair miles before he would let me park in a handicapped space. He'd say, "That's handicapped. I'm not handicapped."

This *overt* type of denial is most often exhibited by a patient. Caregivers tend to express *covert* types of denial, typified by the refusal to educate themselves or to attend support groups or to take safety precautions for their spouses. This is commonly seen in families dealing with Alzheimer's disease, where the impaired person is still allowed to use the stove or to work with potentially dangerous electrical or mechanical equipment.

I shouldn't need to point out how destructive denial can be. But denial can also can work in positive ways. Those like Arthur, for instance, who deny that they have a terminal illness, often keep fighting longer and harder than those who give up and let the illness take over:

> One of the things that drives me is that I'm scared of dying. I really don't want to die. At some point I know I will, but while intellectually it's easy to come to grips with that, emotionally it's not. So I have probably been in that classic first denial step for ten years now, and that's perhaps not the worst thing in the world. I refuse to admit to myself that I really am that sick.

But Arthur must walk a very fine line. Even while keeping a positive attitude and refusing to give in to an illness that he has been told is terminal, he must acknowledge the disease enough to seek out proper medical treatment:

> One of the dangers is that because I don't really accept that I am that ill, I will put everything off until it is too late. But I think my attitude is probably what's making the difference, the reason I'm still here. I think it's a very positive force.

There was a positive side to Michael's denial, too. During his five-week stay in the hospital when he lost his second leg, the doctors told me that this was it. Nothing in his body worked. His kidneys had failed, his heart was damaged, and his circulation was almost nonexistent. He wouldn't recover. He would lie there until he weakened and died.

Michael refused to give in to that verdict. He came home and *lived for another year*, and then his doctors became the ones who were amazed. "I have never met a man who was more in control," one of them later told me. "He had a will that was unbelievable. He had the most invincible will I've ever encountered in a person. His attitude made all the difference, and there is no way he would have lived another year without it."

Today Is Forever

My entire mental attitude, too, was a form of denial. It was vital that I make Michael believe that I believed, with all my heart, that he had a long life to live. In order to do that, I had to believe it too.

What I believed was that he would make it through this current crisis and live at least two more years. But I said for myself to hear, and to anyone who asked, that he would live somewhere between twenty minutes and two years. I did that so I wouldn't be completely overwhelmed if he died the next day. But his stubbornness and will and determination eventually gave me the absolute conviction that he would last the two years.

If I had mentally said to myself, "He's not going to last very long, so I had better start preparing myself emotionally and financially, better tell the children, better restrict myself to short-term business deals," he never would have believed that he could live, because *he would have felt the doubt in me.*

I approached practical matters from the same point of view, making the changes in the house, getting nursing help, and taking day-to-day steps to make a long-term scenario bearable. By opening my eyes to the realities of long-term caregiving, much down-the-road hardship, both financially and emotionally, was averted.

I treated Michael as though he would live forever. I knew he wouldn't, but I knew he would live long enough that I had to treat it as though it would be forever. Had I treated it as a temporary thing and had he then lived for several years longer than I anticipated, I could have become very depressed with the eternal toil of it, because it certainly wasn't any fun.

In order to plan for forever, I bought all the equipment we needed for Michael. I could have rented a lot of it, but I had to buy it in order to convince myself and him that we would be needing it for a long time. This was perhaps impractical from a financial standpoint, but *because it made him believe that he would live,* it was worth it to me.

In addition, I was always planning something for us to do. That had been true even before Michael got sick, but once he was down, it became more important than ever because it gave him *something to look forward to.* And it was important that the initiative was taken by me. I never asked, "Do you want to do such and such?" or "Shall we have Faye and Bob over?" which would have given him an easy out. I simply made continual plans to go somewhere, to invite people over, and I would invite someone for dinner a month ahead of time instead of tomorrow, which would have implied that we were running out of time. I planned as though we were dealing with an abundance of time, that there was unlimited time stretching ahead of us.

In a long-term battle with chronic illness, you usually feel like you're sliding backward. But even in the worst scenarios there are temporary plateaus, and it's important to recognize these, to accept them as the best that's going to be right now, and to enjoy the breathing room. Again, that means adjusting your attitude. And, as I hope I have shown, attitude *can* be changed by reaching out and taking positive action. *The only requirement is that you have to want to do it.*

I never had a Pollyanna attitude. I never acted as though everything were going to be all right. But I was very positive. If you *believe* that things will get better, they will, if only in your mind. And your mind is what this book is all about.

BEAR IN MIND:

Learn and control a positive attitude. With chronic illness you've got to mourn what's lost, but you also need to understand what's still there.

Don't get sad—get mad!

Plan something that will focus your thought process outside yourself and your own problems.

Give yourself to others besides your spouse. There is a difference between giving out of necessity and giving because you want to.

Educate yourself. Knowledge is the key to control.

Treat your spouse as though he or she will live forever.

11
Getting on with the Rest of Your Life

Nearly all patients and caregivers reach a point when they decide to make the most of their lives within the limitations of the illness involved. Perhaps Frank, who has had non-Hodgkin's lymphoma since 1983, describes it best:

> There's a point where you lock on, a point where you say, "I'm going to give this thing all I've got." The quality of life is not the same, but it's good enough.

For the patient, "locking on" can mean the difference between life and death. For the caregiver it can mean the difference between a life that is nothing more than mere existence and one that is a rich and full experience.

Vanessa and Dennis have a five-year-old daughter, Heather. Two weeks before her birth, Dennis had a cerebral aneurysm that changed the structure of the marriage, and of the family, forever. Vanessa explains the difference between what her life could look like and what she chooses to make of it:

> I'm thirty-five years old, a young woman. I have such potential for so many things, and I look ahead at my life and I see that I'm married to someone still in his thirties who's turned sixty-two and frail overnight.

185

We're never going to get to bicycle through the south of France. I haven't lived a full life yet. I'm still raring to go, and I sometimes look ahead and think, "What's in it for me?" But instead of wallowing in self-pity, I decided that when Heather is thirteen or fourteen, she and I will bicycle through France together. Dennis can meet us in Paris.

The Moment of Acceptance

Both Vanessa and Frank have accepted their changed circumstances, although not quickly and not without pain. In many ways their attitude reminds me of the way Elisabeth Kübler-Ross described terminal patients' acceptance of their coming death. "It is as if the pain had gone, the struggle is over. . . [T]he circle of interest diminishes," she wrote in her landmark book, On Death and Dying.

Chronic illness brings a death of sorts. It is the death of health and independence, of the life that once was led, and of the normal, healthy relationship two people once enjoyed. When patient and caregiver accept these losses, the pain of denying the presence of the illness, of railing against it in anger, or of being depressed by it is lessened considerably and sometimes even disappears. The struggle against acknowledging the limitations it imposes goes away. Patient and caregiver do not lose interest in the outside world, but *instead of focusing on what they can no longer do, they concentrate on what is possible.*

So often patient and caregiver are able to pinpoint the distinct moment when their attitude turned from one of struggle, resentment, and anger to one of acceptance. Often it had to do with a return of their feelings of self-worth.

Sometimes this renewed feeling of self-worth comes with the realization that the illness can be managed, that patient and caregiver now know what to expect. Consider Cynthia, who has lupus:

You go through a period where you feel you have to tell people that there's something wrong with you, but I don't feel the need now to talk to someone about my condition every single day or mention the fact that I have lupus. I think it probably took me two or three years to get to the point where I feel like I am living with the disease rather than having the disease run my life as it did in the beginning.

As often as not, what brings about the moment of acceptance appears to have little to do directly with any stabilization or improvement in the illness. It seems to come instead with the introduction of a new possibility, something that leads patient and caregiver to look at themselves and their situation in a different way. Frank's wife, Ann, recalls their moment:

The person who got Frank turned around was this neat little resident from Australia. Frank asked him if he was going to be disabled. He looked at Frank and said, "What kind of job do you have?" Frank told him the name of the company he worked for. He asked, "Do you sit at a desk?" Frank said yes. Then the resident said, "Well, you're sitting in this bed, aren't you? You can do at a desk whatever you can do in this bed."

I did not know about this moment of acceptance for most of the time that I was caring for Michael. I do believe, however, that I unwittingly brought it about for him by creating a situation in which he could view himself in a highly positive light. I have come to call it "Mike's Night."

The Genesis of Mike's Night

The idea that eventually grew into Mike's Night came to me shortly after I brought Michael home from the hospital after he'd lost his second leg. He was unconscious at first, and I had to employ round-the-clock nursing care. Two weeks later he was nicely regaining his strength, but there was one enormous problem: he had lost the will to live, lost interest in the world beyond his own sickness and suffering.

All along people had been calling me at work and asking me about Michael. Now I began to encourage them to call him instead of me. As I saw it, this served three purposes: it showed Mike that people cared about him, it kept him busy, and it made his friends and business associates aware that he was still Mike—the mind, the personality, the things that made him uniquely himself were still there. I'd guide them as to what to say: "Call Mike and let him know how things are at work," or "Call Mike and get his opinion on that." I'd urge them to think about stopping by to visit him. But the depression over his situation continued to haunt our lives.

It was obvious that all of these people cared for Michael, but they didn't know what to say or do to show it. The thought came to me that perhaps some vehicle could be created to help them express what they were feeling, that if Michael realized how much they cared, perhaps he could begin to peer out of the pit he was in and begin to take an interest in life once again. That's when the idea came to me: "I know. We'll give him a party!"

Bear in mind that Michael was still very ill at this point, totally dependent and with full-time nursing care. When I presented my idea to Cox Broadcasting, where he was still a senior vice-president, the reaction was, "My God, you've got to be kidding!" I wasn't kidding.

I knew that Michael would not accept a "party" party, with people getting together to say, "Nice Michael." His pride would not allow that. What he could accept, though, was a roast, where people got up and insulted him in a spirit of fun. And he could accept it even better if he knew it was for a good cause.

Michael's boss at Cox, Bill Schwartz, agreed to the idea and offered to have the company coordinate the party as a benefit for the Diabetes Association. We would create a roast for Michael on his birthday. It would be a *surprise* party. We would charge $150 per person with proceeds going to the American Diabetes Association Georgia Affiliate, Inc.

Planning Mike's Night

We were none of us sure, when we began planning Michael's party, whether or not he would live to attend it. This was a concern that hung in the air unsaid until it threatened to undermine the entire project. I thought it might help to bring it out into the open, to make light of it so others could deal with it. "We need to go ahead and get started with the planning," I began saying. "If Michael doesn't live for this, he's going to be in big trouble." That eased the tension.

We had decided on a surprise party because we were afraid that if we told Michael, he might veto the whole idea. But we felt he needed *something* to look forward to as he gained strength, and we needed to create a diversion to cover any inadvertent slips we might make, so we came up with a decoy event. Michael's boss called and told him that some of his friends at Cox wanted to celebrate his birthday with a small dinner party and that he was expected to be there. When Michael hung up the phone, I innocently asked what the call was about. Keeping a straight face at that moment was a fun part of the game that was beginning to give me a huge lift.

The planning had a similar effect on everyone involved. There was so much to be done: invitations had to be sent, the program planned, things sneaked from the house (like old pictures for montages and old address books for contacts). It became a major business project. Two vice-presidents at Cox, John Furman and Pat Gmiter, took charge. Many of the people who worked on putting together Mike's Night referred to that work as a labor of love.

As the date for the party approached, Michael began

coming to the office once or twice a week, driving a car with hand controls. There was so much going on about the party that the guard at the gate had to notify us every time Michael drove up so people could hide whatever they were working on. The fact that the party was supposed to be a surprise eluded a number of invited guests. They sent letters addressed to Michael saying, "Sorry I can't make your surprise party." The secretaries intercepted them. Because people had been so frustrated by not knowing what to do to help Michael, the planning became a kind of mission for everybody involved. One of the secretaries told me, "I have never in my life worked on anything as fulfilling as this."

And then Michael began having physical complications. He was on dialysis twice a week and was afraid he would have to have surgery on his hands. His doctors, who had been involved with the party from the very beginning, tried valiantly to stave off any worse problems. Michael's second prosthesis had been ordered, and I asked his doctor to expedite its manufacture. Although Michael wouldn't have the strength or healing to stand on it, I knew that it would mean a lot to him to be able to give the appearance of having two legs.

Mike's Night

Tuesday, April 7, dawned—and remained—a beautiful day. We had sent out five hundred invitations and expected maybe one hundred people to show. To our surprise, we had *two hundred and fifty paid attendance* from all over the country, including one friend who had to come from Paris. At 6:00 P.M., the eighteen people invited to the "dinner party" assembled on an upper floor of the Hyatt Ravinia for a small cocktail reception. Invitations to the roast directed the other guests to a ballroom on the main level and instructed them to arrive promptly at 6:30 P.M. and refrain from using hotel elevators between 5:45 and 6:15. Every detail was planned. Michael and I were running late as usual, and I drove like a speed demon down the highway in order to fit our elevator ride into that small window of time. He wondered aloud what my hurry was about.

Michael's intuition had been telling him there must be something bigger in the works, so when we got to the reception he seemed a little disappointed to learn that was all there was. After about an hour we got a call that dinner was ready downstairs. That was our cue. We got onto the elevator to head for the ballroom and Michael's real party. Midway down, one of the out-of-town guests stepped in and we stared at each other in a moment of sheer shock. Fortunately we both recovered quickly, and I asked her if she was in town to visit her father. She said yes and got off hurriedly at the next floor. The rest of us breathed a collective but quiet sigh of relief.

We got off on the main floor and went around the corner to the grand ballroom. *It was filled—with what seemed like virtually everyone Michael had ever known in his life.* They sang and cheered. Flashbulbs popped. Michael looked around with his mouth gaping open. He saw his sister. He saw his friend Ray who had come from California. He saw the friend who had come from Paris. He saw one of his children. He saw a group of colleagues. He began to sob.

He didn't want to shake hands because his were wrapped in bandages, so everyone bent down and hugged him instead. They smiled and cried simultaneously, thrilled to be a part of it all.

Five or six roasters took their turns poking fun at Michael. Two hours after the celebration had begun, with everybody full and tired, with the birthday cake cut and eaten and the singing over, we handed the microphone to Michael. He spoke beautifully as he told these many people who loved him that in the hospital he had drawn his strength from them. He described what it was like getting out and discovering that he didn't know what had happened to the last five weeks of his life. He'd been an actor in his youth and had appeared in several Hollywood movies, and it was as if his actor self had come back. He was composed. His command was extraordinary.

Finally he said, "I don't know whether I'll ever be able to stand up again—much less walk—for the rest of my life. But I want you to know I'm going to try—and I'm going to do it . . . right . . . NOW!"

He put the microphone down. You could hear a pin drop. Then he *stood up!*

The place went wild. Even the waiters and waitresses sobbed. People screamed and cheered, even guests who'd never known Michael. I closed the evening with a prayer, the party broke up, and everyone flowed over to hug Michael again.

It was an unbelievable night. I felt like there was nothing else I could ever do in my whole lifetime that would equal this. I knew I had seen the moment when Michael decided he was going to live.

For the rest of his short life Michael was able to draw on the strength he'd marshalled on Mike's Night, because *he knew people loved him as he was, not just for what he had been.* And the party was important not only for him but also for all his friends and colleagues. They'd been given a chance to let him know in person that they cared, rather than having to wait until he died and then say, "If only I had done something while he was alive." There are so many things that happen to make friends feel bad when someone they love is hurting—seeing their pain, not being able to help—that if we can create something to make these people feel good, it's worth everything.

As for me, the moment I accepted my situation as caregiver to a spouse who was chronically ill had come a year earlier, the week I ran away to Grand Cayman Island and realized I had to put my prized new business venture on hold and begin rebuilding my life with a different set of priorities. Sometime during the early stages of planning Mike's party, however, I experienced a new stirring of hope. I believed I was the only one who could make Michael turn around, because he didn't have it left in him to do it himself. Getting him back on track became my priority. *After* the party was going to be my time. I felt that he would understand, and he did.

Planning Your Own Celebration

It is not the scale of Mike's Night but the spirit of it that is important. That is something anyone can duplicate. You can honor your loved one who is chronically ill and give that person's friends, family, and colleagues an opportunity to express their friendship and love. It doesn't have to be a big party in a hotel ballroom; you don't have to invite five hundred people. You can organize something as simple as a summertime picnic or a gathering of friends in a church fellowship hall. If you heed the following suggestions, you can celebrate your loved one for a very small amount of money and a minimal expenditure of your time:

1. *Be creative.* The best way to be creative, I've found, is to bounce ideas off a few other people and encourage their thoughts on the subject. Have a brainstorming session.
2. *Remember that you're taking a risk.* The patient might not accept or go along with your idea. That's one big reason you need to discuss it with other people who know both you and your spouse very well—children, coworkers, close friends.
3. *Involve an association* if you can. All associations use events as fund-raisers. Contact your local chapter of the association for whatever disease your spouse is suffering from and ask if they can give you an idea of some event you can plug into as a fundraiser in honor of your spouse. You might be talking about a marathon or a bicycle race. Associations are used to planning small events like this in a community, usually charging $5 or $10 per person.
   The best part of involving an association is that the people running it often take care of most of the work of staging the event. They come up with the

idea and do the work, knowing they're going to benefit from the money that is raised, so as an already overburdened caretaker you're not taking on an additional load. Don't be shy about calling. Associations are always on the lookout for ways to become involved with people in the community, because each time they do it opens up a new pool of potential donors and volunteers. It's a win-win situation.

4. *Coordinate the event yourself*—then delegate the planning. That way you do even less work. Based on the experience I had with Mike's Night, the people who did the planning got the greatest reward. They loved it, and it was something they could contribute.

5. *Surprise the person* if you possibly can. And create a subterfuge event by saying you're arranging something smaller—an evening at a friend's house or someone coming over to your house for dinner.

6. *Expect resistance.* The patient will most likely say, "No, I don't want to do it," if the event is not a surprise. If this happens, say, "It's OK if you don't want to come, but we're going to have this anyway." The patient is likely to relent. Still, to avoid disappointment and stress, try for the surprise.

7. *Expect that despite all the extraordinary benefits that may come from such an event, you will almost certainly be depressed afterwards.* A letdown response is normal after any big event. The patient may now be motivated to accept his or her situation and move forward, but life still goes on in its ordinary way, and you may find yourself temporarily wondering whether your celebration really meant anything in the long run. With a little time and patience, however, you will almost certainly find this question answered in the affirmative.

Accepting a chronic illness and the limitations it brings

to both patient and caregiver does not bring joy. But it can bring hope—and *moments* of joy—in a life that is lived with dignity and in as fulfilling a manner as possible. Taking into consideration that all things are relative, it is not farfetched to think of such a life as good.

BEAR IN MIND:

So often patient and caregiver could pinpoint the distinct moment when their attitudes changed from those of struggle, resentment, and anger to acceptance.

You can honor your loved one by giving that person's friends, family, and colleagues an opportunity to express their friendship and love.

PART II
THE PRACTICAL
SIDE

12
Doctors and Hospitals

W hen someone in your family is sick for a long period of time, doctors and nurses become auxiliary family members, and hospitals become your second home. It is therefore crucial that you know how to interact with medical personnel. Because many of the people we talked to hadn't yet learned this important skill, there was a prevailing sense of anger toward doctors and nurses. Much of this aggravation can be alleviated by educating yourself about the illness, by understanding hospital procedure, and—most important of all—by getting the best doctor you can find and then communicating with him or her in an effective manner.

The Quarterback

The medical group that Michael and I dealt with was large, consisting of twenty-five or thirty doctors plus nurses and clerical staff. The letterhead was a little intimidating, but included in the long list of names was "our" doctor. In our minds he became the head doctor. It didn't matter what was wrong with Michael at any specific time; he was the doctor to whom we turned. He made himself available twenty-four hours a day and made Michael and me feel that we could call him at any time if we needed him. If he was going out of town, he made sure we knew who was in charge and he gave us that person's home phone number if we were at a crisis point.

He was our Quarterback, and I turned to him whenever I became desperate. On several occasions when Michael was in the hospital, things were in a state of confusion and I had a sense that nobody was in charge. It was most likely a Saturday afternoon when a lot of interns were running around and no key doctors were on duty. Instead of panicking, I called our Quarterback. "Doctor, we have a potential problem here," I'd tell him. "I need you to take over."

Choosing the Right Doctor

How do you go about choosing your Quarterback? Before beginning the search, take the time to assess your needs so that you know exactly what you are looking for.

Before your spouse became ill, you probably had an internist or family practitioner. Everyone should have a family doctor, a generalist who deals with all types of problems and refers you to specialists if necessary. Most people find this type of doctor through word of mouth—by talking to friends and neighbors. What they want is someone they like and, more importantly, someone they trust.

When a husband or wife becomes chronically ill, your needs change. Your family doctor will not necessarily be the best qualified person to deal intricately with one specific disease over a long period of time, especially if your spouse is going to require a substantial amount of long-term, specialized medical care. The next step, then, is to find the right physicians for dealing with the particular illness. Your goal now is to find the best, and by that I mean the person or persons who are tops in their field. Steve, whose wife has heart disease, did not pussyfoot around on this issue:

> You cannot hesitate to get the very best help. I'm not one to shop around for the best deal. I want to know who's the very best, and I'll find that person.

Doctors have reputations, and a good way to find the best is to ask around within the medical community. If you are looking for a cardiologist, don't ask your neighbor whom he sees for his ulcers. *Ask a medical professional.* Start with your family doctor and ask, "Is there someone else we could call in?" or "Could you recommend a specialist who would be the very best?" Get two or three names. Some people will even go a step further and ask another doctor, cross referencing until the same name or names begin showing up on everybody's lists.

Once you have pinpointed the best specialists, it's time to interview them. Start with a phone call to their receptionists. Say that you are looking for a doctor for your husband or wife, and ask whether he or she could spend a few minutes talking with you about medical philosophy and methods of treatment. This can be done over the telephone, or you can schedule an actual appointment. You may be charged for an office visit, but the price of a half-hour consultation or two should be well worth the cost if the end result means getting the best available medical care.

What you are looking for is someone you can work with over a long period of time. Does he or she talk to you and your spouse as equals? Will all tests and procedures be explained in advance and all thinking be shared every step of the way? Do you feel that the person cares about your family in a genuine way? Is he or she aware of the importance of working with the family as a unit?

It takes a certain kind of physician to interact positively with your spouse and with you. A doctor can be technically brilliant, but without an understanding of some of the emotional things going on in your family he or she is absolutely no good to you and in some cases can actually aggravate your spouse's condition by keeping everyone in a state of upset.

Bedside manner—the manner in which a physician interacts with patients—is an important enough quality that a doctor with a particularly good one can routinely discharge patients from the hospital several days sooner than another one might, just because he or she is skilled at making them feel good about themselves. But bedside manner extends further than the bed. It encompasses communication, warmth, and compassion.

An example of good bedside manner that didn't take place anywhere near the hospital bed was exhibited by Ed's doctor. After a cancer battle that included having every organ in his body biopsied, Ed developed a small polyp in a sinus. It needed to be biopsied, but for Ed that represented the last straw in a two-year fight, and he refused to have it done. Instead of chastising him, the doctor said, "I understand where you're coming from. It would be better if we knew right now, but if we know in a month, that'll be OK, too." With the pressure off, Ed eventually went in.

The type of bedside manner required depends on the type of illness and the needs of the patient. Dede has lupus. She was hospitalized during the initial bout, but she is now controlling her disease at home and has few crisis situations:

> My doctor doesn't have the world's best bedside manner, but on the other hand I don't feel that I need that. If I depended a lot on somebody's having the time to talk and hold my hand, I might have had to look further. But I haven't felt that I needed that. Certainly I know that he's available if it's really urgent.

There are other instances, often in times of crisis, when a good beside manner drops a little in importance. You might be willing to overlook a cold or abrasive personality, for instance, if surgical skill is what you need. Again, the choice is yours to make.

When choosing specialists, we always spoke with the person most highly recommended by our Quarterback, and if we liked him or her we stopped the search then and there. If we had any reservations, we continued interviewing until we found someone who satisfied our needs.

Changing Doctors

What if you already have a doctor but you want to make a change? Of Michael's team of doctors, there were three whom I absolutely loved. One was the vascular surgeon, who had been recommended by the Quarterback as the best such specialist around. He was wonderful. He had one of those soft, reassuring voices that puts everyone at ease even in the midst of crisis. That kind of manner is important if you are dealing with an illness that has frequent, severe downswings. A close friend and business colleague of Michael's wanted to make sure that we had the best doctor available, so on his own he made several calls around the country. Each person he spoke with affirmed that the doctor we already had was the best. Had it not been so, we would have made a change.

Some people think they can't change physicians, that they are forever stuck with the first one they see. Nothing could be further from the truth. People change doctors all the time, and a good doctor will even help a patient make the break if there is something lacking in the doctor-patient relationship. A good doctor knows that if he or she and the patient can't work together, the illness can't be fought as best it might.

Getting over your inertia might take a little effort. Sarah's husband was admitted to the hospital as an emergency patient, and she was told that he wouldn't live more than a week without immediate surgery. She had little time to conduct a search for "the best," but realized that she must try because she had no confidence in the surgeon assigned to her husband in the emergency room:

It is very difficult to make a change. It takes a lot of energy. The current situation may be horrible, but the change is more threatening. Sometimes the unknown is so scary that even though the present situation may be terrible, you are afraid to make a change or even look elsewhere for additional help.

Sarah made the effort, made the change, and is certain that her husband is alive because of it.

Sometimes you are satisfied with the doctors you have, but fate decrees that you must move to another city. The same choosing procedure works well, and it can be initiated from your old residence even before you get to the new city. This is what Richard did:

> When we moved back to Pittsburgh, I went back to Cathy's doctor and said, "Give me three or four names of doctors in our vicinity whom you would consider the cream of the crop." Then I went to Cathy's surgeon and asked him the same thing. Out of the four names that he gave me, two were on the first doctor's list, so I went after those two. It just takes a little research.

Whatever your scenario, when choosing doctors *your goal is to find somebody you trust.* If he or she is knowledgeable, can give you good advice, and clicks with you emotionally, then you can be satisfied with whatever course of action is recommended. When dealing with chronic illness, your Quarterback is the most important person on the team. You must keep looking until you find him or her.

Getting a Second Opinion

There are times when it is advisable to get a second opinion. If your spouse is facing a major surgical procedure, for example, and isn't in a state of immediate crisis, you may want to consult with someone else if for some reason you are not satisfied with just one doctor's recommendation.

Some people complain that their doctors seem threatened by the mention of a second opinion. There could be several reasons for that. One might be a result of the way you express yourself. If you don't want to believe what you've been told or if you come across as belligerent or skeptical of the doctor's knowledge, any doctor would bristle. Try to phrase your request in a polite manner—"Is there someone else we could consult with?"—rather than demanding to see a different physician.

Another reason a doctor might balk at the "second opinion" request is that medicine is not an exact science but rather more of an art. There are often many ways to treat a particular problem, and none of them is necessarily the only way. Your doctor expects you to have faith in him or her and to follow the advice you are given. You could go to one doctor after another until eventually you found one who would prescribe a treatment more in line with your own way of thinking, but that doesn't necessarily mean that the first doctor was wrong; he or she just gave different advice. And the risk you run in seeing too many different physicians is that you will search until you find one who tells you what you want to hear, and what you want to hear isn't always the best medical advice.

A physician who has a sufficiently open mind, who is willing to accept second opinions and willing to have his or her decisions put to scrutiny, is probably a good physician. If the doctor you are dealing with is truly upset by your mention of a second opinion and is unwilling to confer with others or to allow you to do so yourself, then you might well be justified in your skepticism.

It Takes Teamwork

"The doctor-patient relationship is one of the keys to success of making things work," says a surgeon. In other words, it's not just the doctor who is going to do the healing; it's the doctor and patient together and often the patient's entire family as well. The educated patient knows this. "The more active you can be," says one, "in the sense of realizing that you're the best judge of how you feel and what's going on, the better the illness can be dealt with."

Rick, a cancer patient, has a particularly good relationship with the professionals who care for him:

> The doctors have been very good with me, and I'm
> very helpful with them. They recognize that I can be
> relatively objective about my condition and that my
> observations will be accurate. They've treated me like
> an adult. Not every doctor does that. Probably the
> reason I'm so comfortable is that they recognize what
> I can and can't do and they treat me accordingly.

Rick's doctors treat him as a responsible, educated patient.
He is perceived that way because he recognized early on
that teamwork was the key to stabilizing his illness.

For the caregiver, *the first step in becoming a part of the
health care team is to educate yourself and your family.* The more
everyone knows about the illness or condition, the more
active a part each person can play in the treatment. Rick's
wife is an equally valuable member of their team:

> A good doctor is willing to look at the value of the
> family's input. I have kept records on Rick. We used to
> keep temperature charts; we used to watch calorie
> intakes, all kinds of things that give the doctors a
> great deal of input so they can make good decisions. I
> worry about some of the people I've seen who don't
> make the effort to handle the tremendous amount of
> data. I wonder how that affects the care of the patient.

Get the whole family involved if you like, but make sure
that if you do, you don't overload the doctor and monopol-
ize his or her time. If ten people call with the same question, any doctor is likely to become annoyed. Arrange a
group meeting with the doctor or appoint a spokesperson
to act as intermediary.

When the issue of removing one of Michael's legs first
came up, I told our Quarterback that we needed to have a
family meeting and asked if he'd be able to find time to join
us. He agreed, so I assembled every family member who

was in town and had the others on standby near a telephone. With Michael there in the room, our Quarterback explained all our options and everything else he had been telling me privately, so that everyone now became a part of the process. There wasn't really a decision to be made because he was the one who had to call the shots, but he made us feel that we had been a part of it.

Getting everyone involved is particularly important when dealing with a chronic illness. A nurse explains:

> You are treating not only the patient; you are treating the whole family. Those family members need to know how to take care of the patient at home. Also, sometimes the patient is so apprehensive that he or she doesn't hear everything. By talking to all of them, the patient gets a much better picture. Having the family there to give support is important.

Chronic illness runs a roller-coaster cycle of ups and downs. This creates a need for pacing when it comes to medical care. When the patient is at a crisis point or on the way to one, you have to know how to reach the doctors twenty-four hours a day. Even if you don't actually call, you need those numbers for peace of mind. Contrary to that is the need to pace yourself when things level out again. Even though you're paying them, doctors should be treated like friends in that when you don't need them desperately you should relax a little, because the illness is going to be going on for a long, long time.

The Importance of Knowledge

With some diseases, such as lupus, damage can be minimized by careful control. If early signs of impending problems are noticed, they can be swiftly dealt with before major organ systems are involved. Cynthia is well aware of this:

It's important to learn as much about your illness as you can; then you learn to live with it a lot better. Some people don't even want to know what they've got. There's no way you can cope with an illness if you don't know what you're dealing with. I firmly believe that if you're given the diagnosis of a chronic disease, you must learn all that you possibly can about it. Learn to live with it rather than having it control your life.

If it doesn't create too much conflict with the nurses, learn to read the charts. In the past, patient records were guarded like top-secret military documents, but recent changes in legislation have established each person's right to information that concerns his or her own body. By picking up the chart each time you visit, you can see what kind of progress took place during the course of the day.

Getting the Doctor's Ear

Sometimes it seems your doctor is too busy to talk to you. Connie Hill, an Atlanta psychologist who runs education classes for the families of Alzheimer's patients, finds this to be a common problem:

> One of their primary beefs is that very often doctors are too busy to sit down and talk with them in detail about what the diagnosis means or how they arrived at it or what the implications are, so they leave the office—just after a major life event has occurred— armed with little or no information.

What many people don't realize is that the problem is not necessarily one of the doctor's purposefully withholding information but probably one of time. Pretend for a moment that you are the doctor. Your schedule is crammed with appointments that hardly give you room to breathe. Into the examining room comes a patient who requires an extra half-hour for discussion about the illness. The whole day is now out of sync, and every successive patient is going to be kept waiting half an hour for his or her appointment. Two such patients, and everyone will be an hour off schedule. All of those waiting will become angry, and you will be blamed.

Doctors are busy; that is a given. So how do you get your doctor to spend time with you? The answer to that is really quite simple—*schedule the time to talk so that it can be budgeted into the day.* When you make your appointment, say that you need some extra time. The receptionist is used to this and will schedule a double appointment. Or mention your need to your doctor, and see what he or she suggests.

Dr. J. Randolf Beahrs of the St. Paul Urologic Surgeons group is typical of many physicians who go out of their way to be accommodating:

> I don't care how long I spend with a patient, but when it compromises another patient, I have a hard time doing it. If you just give me a little warning that you would like a little more time and get it budgeted into my day, then I will do anything. We can schedule a double appointment, you can call me at the end of the day, or I can call you at home. I will always fit you in.

If you are considerate of the doctor, the doctor will be considerate of you. This shouldn't be too difficult to remember if you can keep in mind that doctors are regular people with normal concerns and feelings. As regular people they also have bad days, just like anyone, so if things aren't going as well as usual on any particular day, stop and think about what might be going on behind the scenes. Dr. Beahrs explains:

> Patients have to understand that doctors have bad days, too. It's nothing personal; they've just had a bad day. I might have been up all night with a patient who finally died, and the first patient of the day calls up and says, "Doctor, I'm having this little problem . . . ,"

and it's tough. I'm not asking people to forgive; they
just need to know that sometimes doctors have a
tough day.

Misplaced Anger

A great deal of anger accompanies any chronic illness—
anger on the part of the patient, the care-giving spouse,
and, indeed, the whole family. Anger is an appropriate
reaction to chronic illness and the changes it wreaks in
people's lives, but much of this anger seems to be mis-
placed. For instance, a caregiver who feels guilty taking
that anger out on the patient might instead fling it at the
medical staff. One caregiver even admits that "the doc did a
good job and got all the cancer," but she still hates him—
presumably simply for being the bearer of bad tidings.

There is often anger at the doctor for being unable to
heal; doctors are not supposed to make mistakes or to
perform procedures that don't work. In addition to serious
asthma, Katy has muscular dystrophy of her vocal cords.
Doctors cut and tied them back in an effort to relieve her
breathing problems, an effort that failed to help and that
destroyed her voice:

> My husband still blames the physicians. They did
> what was right, but he has to be angry at somebody
> so he's diverted all his anger to them. He still thinks
> everything is their fault.

Of our whole medical team, there was one doctor whom
Michael didn't like. His bedside manner left something to
be desired, and that gave Michael license to vent all his
frustrations and anger over the upcoming amputation onto
this doctor. The subject matter was part of the problem—if
he'd been the Prince of Wales Michael wouldn't have liked
him because he was associated with such a painful loss—
but his bedside manner made it impossible for Michael to
even try. He was a fine surgeon, though—the best, we

were told—and so we put our personal feelings aside and agreed to let him do the job.

Nurses are easy to blame for anything that goes wrong because they are the most convenient targets, and they often take the brunt of the family frustration. Michael either liked a nurse or hated a nurse. If he hated him or her, he yelled, and I had to learn to look beyond the immediate problem to realize that he was probably in pain or just feeling bad. I always made sure to smooth things over as best as possible if he had been yelling at someone, because—like the nurse or not—we were still dependent on him or her.

Most of this anger stems from loss of control. When illness strikes, life is no longer a play to be choreographed at will. Instead, it resembles a vehicle out of control, rushing headlong down a tunnel with no one in the driver's seat. For the patient the terms of the trip are dictated by pain, fatigue, and dimming physical abilities. For the caregiver the terms are dictated by the endless needs of another person. For the children, joy and fun disappear and are replaced by gnawing fear and unhappiness.

Health-care professionals are beginning to recognize the need to give patients and their families as much control over their lives as possible, the aim being to increase their independence and consequently their enjoyment of life. This can be achieved by giving more and more treatment at home and by being as flexible as possible with therapy administered at the hospital. Kathy Newman, a nurse who administers chemotherapy to cancer patients, explains:

> The most important thing we try to impart to these people is that they can live with cancer. We try to adjust the therapy to their lifestyle so that they can maintain a little control over their lives. If there's a child's birthday party or a family wedding, if they don't feel good or emotionally can't take it, we can change things. That increases their independence, their enjoyment of life. It gives them control. It's so

much better for everyone involved when they're not
stripped of the things they enjoy.

Maintaining Control

I believe that I always have choices—which means that I
have control. In the case of the doctor Michael didn't like,
the choices were going to a doctor with a better bedside
manner but less surgical skill, or making an attempt to get
more from this one. Since the skill was what we wanted,
we opted for the latter, and we eased the situation a little
by having our Quarterback ask the surgeon to administer
just a little more TLC.

What are other ways of maintaining control and thereby
feeling less like a passenger on a speeding vehicle? First of
all, try to analyze the source of your anger. Is the problem
really the doctor, or is it simply the loss of control that
makes the situation so unbearable?

Ralph's wife was in the final stages of cirrhosis when he
took her in to see her physician. They sat in the waiting
room for two hours before Ralph took it upon himself to
ask the receptionist how much longer the doctor would be.
When told that the doctor had been at the hospital dealing
with an emergency, Ralph exploded. "Do you mean to tell
me that Margaret has been sitting out here in a metal chair
for two hours and the doctor hasn't even left the hospital?
We're gone!" Two years later he is still fuming about that
incident because his wife died before getting back for her
rescheduled appointment.

To avoid such situations with Michael, I made sure I was
introduced to and knew by name my Quarterback's two
primary office nurses. In the office every day of the week
was a roomful of waiting people, and there was no way
that Michael, in severe pain, was able to sit there with
them. Knowing that doctors aren't usually available to
come to the phone during a busy day, I would call these
nurses and say, "Michael is hurting badly. I need to bring
him in. When is the best time? Could you check with the

doctor and get right back to me?" Making friends with the assistants is like making friends with a secretary—it smooths the path for any action you need to take.

The nurses knew that Michael would come in only if he was desperate. When we arrived, they immediately took him into an empty room, put him onto a bed, and gave him an injection so that he would be relaxed and in less pain by the time the doctor came in.

If I had to take him to the emergency room I did the same thing. I had the nurses or the doctor call ahead to let the staff know we were coming. When we arrived they already knew Michael's history, and they could usually deal with him without having our doctor come in.

Regaining Control in Nonemergency Situations

- Ask for a meeting with the key people—the doctor and the head nurse, for instance.
- Write down the issues you are going to cover so that you come across in a rational, businesslike manner rather than as an enraged spouse. You will be more in control if you commit your feelings to paper.
- Cushion your anger, hostility, or fear with phrases like, "It seems like . . ." or "I realize it may not be the case, but I feel like . . ."
- Make a list of what you would like to see corrected and hand it over to the appropriate person.
- Keep a copy of the list so that you can follow up.
- Acknowledge progress with a simple "thank you."
- When the problem is fixed, send a written note of gratitude.
- As a last resort, ask your doctor about the feasibility of changing hospitals.

We did change hospitals a couple of times, although not because of any problems with staff; I just thought that it might help Michael psychologically if he could have a change of environment. Since he only went into the hospital if something bad happened, he had nothing but negative associations with his regular hospital, and the mere drive to it was enough to sink him into a deep gloom. I thought that a change of staff, a different view out the ·vindow, might be of help.

I was insistent on the selection of hospitals for other reasons, too. One reason I was so happy to have Michael home was that the hospital where his group practiced was a good forty-five minutes from our house and was in a difficult part of town to go through by myself at night. After some time I began insisting on going to a closer hospital if all we were doing was going in for tests and as long as it didn't compromise his care. This may seem at first like a selfish consideration, but when you are dealing with an illness that will require you to make that trip hundreds of times, it's no light matter. For us it became an even larger issue after we moved another thirty miles away and Michael began requiring dialysis several times a week. I then requested that the doctors explore every possibility within a fifteen-minute radius of our new house.

When Michael was transferred to one particular hospital, we learned an astonishing fact: the bathrooms in the hospital rooms did not accommodate wheelchairs. Michael decided to do something about that, not for his stay but for other patients in the future. He wrote a letter to his doctor and to the hospital administrators, and as a result his recommendations were made a part of the upcoming renovation plans. That gave him a great sense of accomplishment—and a feeling of once again being in control.

Assessing Tests and Procedures

A number of interview subjects expressed anger at physicians for prescribing unnecessary or expensive tests and procedures. While most doctors don't recommend any tests that aren't in their opinion necessary for the diagnosis and treatment of the patient, things do occasionally get out of control—particularly when many different physicians are involved with one case. To compound the problem, some people are so intimidated by the medical profession that they let themselves become pawns in the hands of the doctors instead of becoming a part of the health-care team.

Cynthia, on the other hand, does not let herself be intimidated by doctors:

> Most people just blindly go in and let doctors do things to them. There are many people out there who are brought up with the mentality that if the doctor says do it, you *must* do it. There are an awful lot of needless procedures done.
>
> Some of the consultants were talking about scheduling what we call "exotic studies." One guy walked into my room one night and said, "We're going to move you to another hospital to do five or six tests." I had just met this man, and I said, "Wait a minute, who made this decision? I'm not going because I don't see any point in it."
>
> He could not believe that a patient was telling him this. He pointed out how ill I was. I said, "I'm sorry, but I just don't let some stranger come in and command control of my life. I need to talk with my husband, I need to talk with my personal physician, and then, if I feel it's necessary, I'll go. But I'm not going just because *you* decided I should go."
>
> My internist agreed with me that these tests were probably not going to do anything except make the doctors feel better. And that's always been the bottom line: if the treatment is going to change and will result in a more beneficial effect for me, then I will go along with it. But if the only reason they're doing it is to make the doctor feel better or make the paper they're filling out look better, then I don't believe in wasting my energy or resources. If it's not going to change the bottom line, why are we doing it?

It takes a sophisticated consumer of medical information to decide whether or not a particular test is necessary. This is another good reason to educate yourself. It's also another reason why good communication with the doctor is so important: if you don't feel that you know enough to make an informed decision yourself, you at least deserve an explanation of the test or procedure and what it will accomplish.

Financial matters also come into play here. The "bottom line" can refer to expense as well as results. Sometimes doctors need to be told that insurance isn't covering all costs, that "exotic studies" are financially out of the question. Barbara, whose husband lost both of his legs and all of their money to diabetes, has a strong opinion on this issue:

> I think that the person who is responsible for the bills should be talked to. For instance, we went to get the prostheses. One prosthesis is $5,000! Two prostheses are $10,000! They are not covered by any of our insurance. The doctor should have taken me aside, I think, and told me what this was going to cost, because $10,000, when you're already in debt $25,000, is something you just don't have. And my husband has only been able to stand up for thirty seconds with his prostheses because he can't use his hands!

Why did the doctor prescribe something that cost so much yet was going to be of so little use? Barbara had a right to know ahead of time, just as you have a right to be informed and to discuss all tests and procedures before they are performed. But the doctor may not go into things in detail unless he or she knows you have educated yourself enough to discuss it.

In the Hospital

Many chronically ill people spend a lot of time in the hospital. Since they are sick even when they are at home, they are generally in real trouble by the time they arrive at the emergency room. Hospital stays are stressful occasions for everyone. The patient is struggling to survive; you and the family are worried; the room is claustrophobic, dark, and uncomfortable. The doctor isn't there when you need him or her, and the nurses seem too busy to help out. What can you do to help?

Probably the greatest contribution you can make to anyone's hospital stay is to make things go as smoothly as possible. There are many ways to do this:

- Give support, but make sure that support is what you think it is. A nurse explains:

  The best thing caregivers can do is give support in a calm and reassuring manner. The worst mistake they can make is to hover over the patient, even to the extent of answering questions asked by the medical staff. They don't mean to do it; they're helpless and scared, and they're trying to help. But what they are doing is compromising that patient's independence.

- Observe and respect what I call the "panic time" of the staff. This is usually at the change of nursing shift—at 7:00 A.M., 3:00 P.M., and 11:00 P.M. Everyone is in a state of frenzy for about forty-five minutes on either side of the bewitching hour. That is not the time to ask for something, but it *is* a good time to visit someone critically ill who might be helpless and in need of assistance.
- Another good time to visit is on the weekend. Weekends in the hospital can be a traumatic experience for someone who is there a lot. There are probably no key doctors around because the A team is off duty and the B team has taken over. The change of nurses is constant.
- I always left on Michael's nightstand the number where I could be reached, but he often moved it

somewhere else and then couldn't find it. I made a habit of giving it to the nurse as well so that if necessary the nurse could place the call for him.

• I did my best for Michael, and I also made an effort to help out the staff as much as possible. One extreme example of this was a time when I hired private-duty nurses to look after Michael just after his two major surgeries. He was so confused (this was a side effect of certain medications) that he did harmful things to himself, such as pulling out his IV or trying to escape, and the regular staff couldn't look after him every minute. On two other occasions when he was quite alert, we actually had to put a big sign on his wheelchair saying "Return this patient to room 305," and once the kids took his clothes so he couldn't leave.

• In order to get the most out of the staff—meaning the best care for Michael—I acted as his public-relations agent. When dealing with chronic illness you must not burn any bridges, because you will be dealing with the same people again and again. I tried my best to be tactful and appreciative, and I did what I could to smooth over any problems Michael had caused.

• I went by the nurses' station daily and introduced myself: "I'm Beverly Kievman. Are you Mr. Kievman's nurse today? How do you think he's doing?" My objective here was to become a person and to make him a person in their eyes rather than just another grouchy face on the pillow.

• Each week I asked Michael's nurse how long he or she would be on duty. If the answer was, "I'll be on this shift all week," I paid more attention to that person. I always wrote down the name so that I knew it whenever I came to visit or had to call. And I did need to call that nurse at times, because during a couple of crisis situations after his surgeries I occasionally phoned Michael and found him delirious.

Sometimes he even dropped the phone, which left me understandably concerned. A quick call to the nurse could reconnect us or, if necessary, summon help.

- Michael had frightening side effects from codeine, but, after surgery, if he was in a confused state and in pain, codeine was sometimes the drug he received. We'd had a terrible problem with this, and I needed to set things up so that it didn't happen again. But instead of coming across like a battle-ax, I made a point of saying to the nurse, "I would like to thank you in advance for looking out for that particular problem because we have had trouble with it before."

- If our favorite nurse had done tough duty, I rewarded that hard work with some of the food or flowers that were in the room. I also gave small gifts to other nurses who had gone out of their way.

Key Phrases for Getting Things Done

- "I'd appreciate your help with . . ."
- "When you have a breather, could you please check . . .?"
- "Anything I can do to help you with (the patient) tonight?"

Circumventing Hospital Routine

Since hospitals are labor-intensive places of work, strict routines have been set up to make things run smoothly. If you are a regular visitor, the routine isn't always easy to live with. I discovered that it can be circumvented, but in order to get around hospital routine, you must first understand it.

If the patient has just missed a meal when checking into the hospital, food can be obtained simply by asking for it. It is also possible, at any hour of the day or night, to order crackers, cookies, ice cream, fruit, or beverages. If Michael wasn't eating well, I had the nurses keep his bedside table stocked with fruit that he could eat if he woke up during the night.

Michael was in intensive care a lot, sometimes for weeks at a time. There were huge visitation-times signs posted, and they were so forbidding that to enter at any but those permitted times appeared as though it would interfere with the world. I quickly learned that wasn't so, that it was possible to visit Michael at times more convenient to me. If I didn't ring the bell and ask to come in but instead quietly opened the door and walked in like I was there on official business, no one ever said anything. I could quietly visit for ten or fifteen minutes and then slip away again. I am by no means trying to incite active rebellion here, because there are important reasons for those limited visits with inten- sive-care patients, but when you are there a lot it some- times pays to work out your own routine—as long as it does not interfere with the staff's responsibilities to your patient and others.

The hospital where Michael spent most of his time had a spectacular view of downtown Atlanta—on one side. The rooms on the other side offered a view of what looked like the tops of steam boilers. If we checked in as an emergency, he was usually given one of the rooms with no view and stuck way down at the end of the hall. On Friday, when many of the other patients had checked out, I always asked to have him moved. Even if he was asleep or so ill that he had no regard for his surroundings, I asked for a room with a view so that when he did feel better he'd be able to enjoy it.

I also asked for a room change whenever he was in a rather critical state. I had him placed as close as possible to the nurses' station so that if he couldn't figure out how to buzz for his nurse, he could yell instead.

I arranged for automatic check-in and checkout. This saves reams of time if your spouse has a condition that sends him or her to the hospital frequently. It can be arranged through the doctor, or you can do it yourself through the admissions office. Drop in, let them know that your spouse is probably going to be a constant patient, and see what can be done to arrange for automatic billing, check-in, and checkout. What you're doing is becoming a person to them. Whenever they see you arrive they say, "Go on up. We'll take care of the paperwork later."

I made myself at home in the hospital room. The chairs for visitors are historically uncomfortable, but I discovered that it is usually possible to obtain a better one. It's worth the small effort, because you'll be spending a lot of time in it.

I brought Michael's pillow along from home, covered in a brightly colored pillowcase. This tiny act served several functions: it made Michael feel at home, it gave the nurses something to comment on, and it made Michael stand out.

I also brought along a couple of photographs. Again, this had more than one function. It gave Michael something to look at, and it made him more of a person in the nurses' eyes. It also gave them a conversational starting point when he was depressed and lethargic.

The nurses always had fresh coffee brewing at their station, and they were usually more than happy to share it with me so I didn't have to go all the way down to the cafeteria. In return, I asked where the ice machine was and kept Michael's ice bucket filled.

While you're waiting for a surgical operation to be performed, you usually find yourself in a dreary, uncomfortable waiting room filled with nervous smokers. If a telephone exists, it is probably good only for incoming calls. There are sometimes rooms available for special situations. Each time Michael was having a life-threatening or critical surgery (like an amputation), our Quarterback arranged for us to have use of a conference room that gave our family some privacy. It even had a phone from which we could make outgoing calls without storing up quarters. There are times when you want to ask for that. If your spouse is undergoing a difficult surgical procedure and it's important that you maintain contact with the rest of the family and that the doctor knows where you are, perhaps you deserve some special consideration, such as a private room for crying, for praying, or for grieving.

Practical Tips

- Before checking out of the hospital, get a starter set of all prescription drugs. If the drugstore is closed or there's a problem on the way home or—and this can actually happen—the local distributor runs out, you are covered for a few days.
- Take any unused supplies home from the hospital, because as soon as a package is opened, you have paid for it.
- Buy commonly used products in quantity, and ask your pharmacy to give you a volume discount. Explain that you are going to be a regular customer, and ask if they are willing to set up a 10 percent discount rate for you. They do for senior citizens, and they might do it for you, too.

Should the Patient Be Told All?

In the not-so-distant past it was common for medical information to be withheld from patients. That attitude has changed, because doctors now recognize the value that knowledge plays in battling disease. Most people nowadays would be outraged to be kept in the dark about things going on in their own bodies. This is how one nurse describes the negative effects of withholding information:

> One thing that irritates me is when the families ask for information to be kept from the patient. People know when something is wrong with their bodies. When family members try to hide things from the patient because they think he or she can't take it,

they're usually masking an inability to talk to each other and with the medical team. That's where we see people hurting so badly—where they're not talking to each other about the way they're feeling.

I believe there are sometimes certain *details* that the patient doesn't need to know, simply because that knowledge won't contribute anything and might actually send the person into a severe depression. My husband was a sixty-three-year-old who looked like a forty-five-year-old, but the doctors told me that he had the insides of an eighty-year-old. Michael didn't need to know that. He had enough to cope with already.

Kathy Newman, who treats many terminally ill patients, understands this fine line between honesty and subterfuge:

> I don't like keeping things from people, although there are rare instances when it's best not to tell somebody something. Sometimes I don't tell someone that they are terminal until they get close to asking me, because where there's life, there's hope. I don't believe in ever, ever, ever taking hope from someone. You must not devastate someone with honesty. That's not in anybody's best interest.
>
> But when it's time to be honest, I can say, as I did to one patient, "Look at what you've accomplished in a year and a half. Look at what you've seen; look how bravely you fought the battles. It wasn't easy: you've been sick and miserable. But you've had some good times, and you've seen your first grandchild. You've fought it the way you wanted to, and now we're going to help you die the way you want to." That is heart-to-heart honesty.

Public Image

Doctors used to have a "Norman Rockwell" image: they stood out in the community as stalwart, conscientious citizens. That image has unfortunately changed, and some people now regard doctors as big egos who are underworked and overpaid, living in big houses and leading the easy life. But that image is misleading. A surgeon explains:

> People just see me as a guy on the golf course and driving a Mercedes. The amount of time I spend caring and giving to patients doesn't get noticed. Today was supposed to be my day off, but I worked all day because I had call after call from patients who needed to be seen. I'm in the business to care for these people, and so I make room in my life to see them. My day gets tromped upon, but no one knows that.

The Mercedes image may not exactly be false, but it doesn't present a complete picture. Doctors do make a lot of money, but before bringing home that large salary they have spent between nine and fourteen years attaining an education. Most are approaching thirty before they begin to earn a full income, and out of that they must pay off educational loans that might run up to $80,000. On top of that expense comes liability insurance that can exceed $100,000 a year—a burden created by us, the public.

As for the "big ego" trait, here's what one doctor has to say about that:

> Doctors need to have a certain ego structure in order to cope with the pressures of practicing medicine, of dealing with life-and-death matters on a daily basis. They need a fair amount of confidence and feeling for what their specialty is in order to be able to practice it, in order to support themselves and support their patients. The doctor's "ego" and the doctor's "pride" are really there for the patient.

Some doctors probably do have inflated egos, just as do some lawyers, some plumbers, some of any group you might look at. If you find yourself dealing with a big ego and it bothers you a lot, remember that you are the consumer. You are paying for a service, and if you don't like any part of what you are getting, you are free to make a change.

Nursing has a different type of public image problem. The image of nursing is not one of a profession; it's more of an occupation, and one that is unfortunately not held in high esteem. This, along with a whole series of other problems such as low pay, inconvenient hours, expense of education, and the availability of more attractive options (such as medical school), is causing a nationwide nursing shortage. The poor image of nursing is even more unfortunate since it comes at a time when nursing skills are becoming more technical than ever before. Nurses are no longer doctors' helpers, and they don't just practice "bedpanology." They monitor high-tech equipment and do far more assessing and thinking than in the past. Contrary to its lagging public image, every aspect of nursing has tremendous responsibilities.

Before becoming too critical of the doctors and nurses you are dealing with, talk to some on a more personal level. Is there a doctor in your neighborhood? He or she will probably welcome a chance to enlighten you. Find out what that life is all about. If you are spending a lot of time in hospitals, chat a little with the nurses. If those who deal with the chronically ill consider getting to know the family a part of their job, then getting to know them a little, too, should be a part of *your* job. Find out how much of themselves they put into their work, how the hours affect their family life, what sacrifices they make for you. You might be surprised at what motivates some of them:

> The nice part of nursing, as compared to medicine, is that you can be with a person for eight hours a day. You get into feelings and hand-holding and touching and all of those important skills. I like working with the whole family.

Doctors also have reasons why they went into medicine and these are usually very interesting reasons, but they don't have the time to tell everyone about them—unless you ask.

The Patient as Consumer

The entire field of medicine is in an enormous state of change. These changes involve every phase of the health-care field. Nothing today is as it was even three or four years ago, and it will not be the same three or four years in the future. You need to examine your choices before choosing physicians, insurance companies, or health-care groups that you could be dealing with for a long, long time.

With the advent of HMOs—health maintenance organizations—and other health-care companies the public has begun to shop around for medical care. All sorts of health-care plans are vying for business, each one offering a "better" deal than the next. If your health care is provided by an employer, you may not have the luxury of a choice of companies and policies; but if you have control over your own health care, try to find a plan that gives you maximum choice in doctors and specialists, even though this may rule out the HMOs. Make sure you're getting the best care, not just the best deal, because your relationship will be a long one.

The field of medicine is more competitive than it used to be; even hospitals are now in the position of having to market their services. That gives you leverage, because administrators are more willing to listen to patients and caregivers than ever before. If you are upset with some aspect of hospital care and request an interview with a hospital administrator, you will most likely get one because the hospital needs your business.

It takes hard work and determination on the part of everyone involved in treating a chronically ill person to make things run smoothly and efficiently. On your part, *the important steps are educating yourself and learning how* hospitals operate so you can get the best possible care for your spouse. *The most crucial step is the choice of your Quarterback.* If you do your homework and get the right person, you should end up as satisfied as Rick:

> We have the greatest doctor in the world. And the reason he's a great doctor is because he's a great human being. He's not defensive; he's not uptight. He's very competent and confident. It makes a big difference.

BEAR IN MIND:

Assess your needs before beginning the search for a doctor.

Don't be afraid to switch doctors. Many people think they are stuck with the first doctor they see.

Find out as much as you can about your spouse's illness and condition. Knowledge is key to control.

Understand the hospital routine.

13
Caring for the Patient at Home

Shortly after Michael died I visited a national trade show for the home health-care industry. It was held at the Georgia World Congress Center in Atlanta, and all of the six hundred forty thousand square feet of exhibit space was devoted to showing the latest in home health-care equipment.

As I wandered up and down the seemingly endless aisles, I found myself increasingly excited—and increasingly deprived. There was wonderful, creative, inventive equipment here. I remember particularly a set of lightweight, portable tracks designed to get wheelchairs over steps, curbs, and other obstacles. They could be carried in the trunk of a car. My mind flashed back to all the wooden ramps we'd had to build, all the buildings Michael couldn't enter, all the experiences that had been denied him simply because we couldn't get his wheelchair up a couple of steps. "Where were these things when Michael was alive?" I asked myself. "Why didn't I know about them when I needed them?"

To me this illustrates part of the dilemma of caring for a chronically ill person at home. There are enormous advantages to home care, yet once the patient leaves the hospital *you* become the Quarterback, and being an effective Quarterback is a learned skill.

228

Learning How to Call the Plays

A good Quarterback carefully studies films of the opposing team to learn what he's up against. He objectively assesses his own strengths and weaknesses and those of his teammates. Only then does he attempt to make the decisions that will hopefully ensure the success of his team. In other words, a good Quarterback learns all he can about what his situation will be come game time. If you plan to take charge of your spouse's home health care, you need to do the same thing, and you need to do it well in advance of the day your spouse is discharged from the hospital or long before an advancing illness requires full-time care.

Start by haunting your local library to find books on home health care and on the specific illness you are dealing with. Most of these books are together in one section, but if years have gone by since you last set foot in a library you may have to ask for help. Many library catalogs are now on microfilm, an easy-to-use system that can at first seem perplexing to anyone who was brought up with card catalogs. It's no crime not to know how to use the new system; we've all had to ask for help at first.

When you've read everything the public library has to offer, go to the nearest university library, particularly if it is connected with a medical or nursing school. Again, enlist the help of the librarian. Allow yourself plenty of time to sit and read since you probably won't be able to check books out, and bring some change for the photocopying machine.

Few of us would select a doctor or a hospital at random, yet that is how many people select a home health-care team, usually because a decision must be made fairly quickly. Don't let time constraints limit your choice, even if it means leaving your spouse in the hospital for another day while you gather information. Do as much groundwork as you can in advance. Check out agencies and equipment dealers. Major decisions—who will care for your spouse, who will supply a wheelchair or oxygen equipment, and so on—should be made only after carefully investigating your available options.

From visiting nurses to equipment dealers to homemakers to your neighborhood pharmacy, your list of providers of outpatient services is almost infinite. Your list of *top-quality* providers, however, is not. Nor is your time. As with the selection of a doctor or a hospital, you will ultimately save time and trouble by familiarizing yourself with the market in advance and shopping around for the best care.

The Home Health-Care Advantage

After Michael lost his second leg and the hospital staff could do no more for him, I knew he would be happier at home. What I did not know was how difficult this would be to manage. As a businesswoman I at least knew the value of establishing a detailed game plan, but when I wandered the hospital corridors I discovered that there was no one who could map out a plan for bringing Michael home. There were doctors, nurses, and social workers willing to answer my questions, but only those questions I thought to ask. What I wanted was a blueprint, but none was available.

In all fairness, even if the hospital had offered me a blueprint, I still would have had much planning to do because no one knew what I did: no one knew our house; no one knew our children; no one knew Michael or me. I was the one who would have to play Quarterback, but I had never played this particular game before.

Taking on this responsibility was stressful, but not nearly so stressful as having Michael in the hospital. Hospitals are in a constant state of flux. Imagine catering a large wedding, a project that takes several weeks to put together. Then imagine you have to deal with a totally new catering staff every day, people who have no knowledge of what the previous day's staff has done. That may give you some idea of what it was like trying to keep track of everyone responsible for Michael's care. What if the morning shift nurse, deluged with patient requests, forgot to fill out a complete patient report for the afternoon nurse? What if a newly assigned nurse, unaware of Michael's terrible reaction to codeine, gave him that as a painkiller?

If I brought Michael home I could place a master list on the refrigerator and more easily monitor who was taking care of him and what medications they were dispensing. There was also a substantial financial advantage. In the hospital, the cost of maintaining expensive medical equipment, mopping the floors, and even taking care of the grounds all figure indirectly into your bill. Since your home health-care team bills you only for those professional or personal services you need as opposed to all of those available, you save money. These are strong arguments for home care. The most powerful, however, is the psychological one. *I wanted to bring Michael home because of the change I knew it would bring about in his attitude.*

A lot has been written about "intensive care syndrome." Patients in intensive care are hooked up to life-support equipment in an environment where there is no day or night. This situation can engender feelings of helplessness, anxiety, and depression. I think something similar can happen even to patients who are not in intensive care if they've been admitted to the hospital a number of times.

I watched it happen to Michael. After he'd been in the hospital half a dozen times, I began to notice that as soon as he checked in he lapsed into what I've come to call his "hospital mentality." Michael never went to the hospital unless he was in intense pain. And here he was again—in pain, in the hospital, back on IVs, back on dialysis, back on medications. Michael's hospital mentality was a survival mode, a totally different mind-set. He became helpless, punctuating his passivity with bouts of anger and hostility as he tried to fight his way through his pain. The anger was his only outlet.

As soon as I brought him home he snapped out of his hospital mentality. He became energized and had a sense of being in control once again. He recuperated faster.

On a more selfish note, I disliked driving to the hospital.

I cannot begin to count the number of times I fought my way through forty minutes of traffic only to discover that Michael had just fallen asleep.

When Michael lost his second leg, I vowed that if there were any way to bring him home, I would do whatever it took.

Smoothing the Transition

No matter what kind of care your husband or wife requires, your key to a smooth transition from hospital to home calls for planning and coordination among (1) your doctor; (2) the hospital staff and discharge planners; (3) the home health-care agency, if you're using one; (4) the equipment dealer, if equipment is needed; and (5) you and your family.

Typically, the responsibility for assuring your mate of follow-up care upon discharge rests with the hospital's office of discharge planning, social services, continuing care, or patient advocacy. Not all of these programs work well, and not all work the same way. Make sure you know how your hospital's discharge planning system is set up and who your contact should be.

Many hospitals rely on a team approach to discharge planning. Beth Israel Hospital in Boston, for example, has a primary care nurse who assumes responsibility for the patient's twenty-four-hour care from admission to discharge. This nurse meets the patient's medical needs by consulting with attending physicians, therapists, family members, and other caregivers. At the same time, he or she plans in advance for the return home. Whether the patient will need a visiting nurse, a homemaker, specialized medical equipment, or community services such as Meals on Wheels, the primary care nurse assumes responsibility for delivering them. As much as possible, the nurse and the staff teach the family bedside techniques such as IV therapy and proper equipment usage.

At nearby Massachusetts General Hospital, in contrast, the patient's nurses, doctors, and social workers meet and produce a discharge plan shortly after admission. A social worker arranges for all required home health-care services before the patient's return home.

Although every hospital employs discharge planning personnel, there is no guarantee that you will see them yourself. Unless otherwise requested, some hospitals limit discharge planning conferences to those patients over a certain age or diagnosed with a particular condition.

Frequently, doctors are unaware of available outpatient services. *Here is where you need to take charge.* Contact the discharge planner yourself, well before your husband or wife is scheduled to return home. This will not only allow that person time to confer with other health professionals and select the best care for your spouse, it will also ease your mind to know that *you are in command of the situation.* In addition, you will avoid the added stress of trying to obtain necessary services at the last minute.

In our case the discharge planner gave us the names of one or two home health-care agencies. The one we chose supplied us with medical equipment, skilled nursing care, and much practical knowledge that I used in caring for Michael.

A wheelchair, a hospital bed, rails for the commode, levers for the faucet—all of these proved helpful. So did knowing how to flush out a temporary dialysis tube, monitor blood sugar levels, and take everyday sterile precautions. The nurses insisted I learn these skills, and they were correct in doing so because there were times when I was the only one available to help Michael. *All caregivers should learn as much as they can about home-care techniques.* If the nurses you hire don't offer to show you, ask them to do so. Most insurance policies do not cover nursing care indefinitely. Learning as much as you can about the nursing procedures needed to care for your loved one will prove vitally important when you are on your own and when the time comes to hire other, nonprofessional help.

Whose Agency Is This, Anyway?

Although Michael and I were both satisfied with our home health-care agency, I would not advise making such an important choice simply because someone at the hospital gave you the agency's telephone number. Find out *who* in the hospital recommends that particular agency and *why*. Take down that person's name and phone number. Mention this person's name when you are talking with the agency. *The key here is accountability.* You are letting the agency personnel know they will be held accountable to this important referral source for the type of care they give your spouse.

Because of changes in Medicare and Medicaid regulations, the current practice is to release patients from the hospital as early as possible. This has created an explosion in the number of agencies supplying home health care. Despite fierce competition for business, services may vary substantially from one agency to the next.

What should you look for in selecting a home health-care agency? To avoid choosing one that cannot fulfill your spouse's needs, familiarize yourself with the company, its background, its personnel policies, and its supervision of employees. A good place to start is with a few pertinent questions. Most of those below were taken from Janet Zhun Nassif's excellent book *The Home Health Care Solution* (Harper & Row, 1985).

Is the company a legitimate home-care agency, or is it instead a nursing registry or employment agency? Be careful. Many registers and employment agencies list themselves in the yellow pages under the same headings as legitimate *home-care* agencies.

Does the agency provide professional references? A reputable agency will supply you with credible references from doctors, hospitals, or community social work personnel. Never settle for the name of a hospital or organization. Insist on names of specific individuals within the hospital or group.

Does the agency limit eligibility for service in any way? Some agencies may limit service to a particular geographic area. Occasionally an agency may provide care only if there is at least one family caregiver in the house or if insurance coverage is available. A public agency such as a county health department may limit service according to income.

Is the agency accredited, Medicare certified, or licensed? Not only does this ensure professional standards, it is a requirement in many insurance policies. Check your policy to be sure.

What is the background of the agency's top management personnel? Management means more than the nurse supervisor. Avoid agencies whose management lacks prior experience in home-care or health-service fields.

Is the agency insured against problems? Although it is an effective advertising gimmick, bonding only protects you against theft. It does not assure you professional service. Professional agencies always carry malpractice and liability insurance.

What services does the agency offer? If it does not provide every service you need, will it help you obtain these services? Not all home health-care agencies supply medical equipment and supplies, and not all home health-care personnel are contractually obligated to perform chore services such as meal preparation. Nonetheless, many of these agencies will arrange for alternative services such as adult day care, Meals on Wheels, and other necessities.

When are the agency's services available? How soon can services begin? Do costs vary depending on the hours worked? Consider the agency's work schedule from the viewpoint of the care you need. I would not recommend entrusting your spouse's care to any agency that cannot accommodate a general request within three business days. You will not want to sacrifice your spouse's care while waiting for a service to begin. On the other hand, round-the-clock service does not necessarily indicate superior quality of care.

As to costs, I was surprised to learn how much more expensive nursing care was on weekends and holidays—you pay time and a half on Saturdays and Sundays, double on holidays. Over Thanksgiving and Christmas I asked our children to lend a hand for a bit of extra money. They were grateful for the additional income, and the arrangement gave Michael some added family companionship that marked these as festive occasions for him.

Can the Health-Care Agency Meet Your Needs?

The services offered by home health-care agencies vary widely in quality and range. To make sure the one you are considering will meet your needs and live up to your expectations, we recommend asking the following additional questions, most of which, again, were taken from *The Home Health Care Solution.*

Does the agency conduct an in-home assessment prior to developing your spouse's care plan and rendering service? No matter how carefully you think you have assessed your own situation, an agency has a professional responsibility to conduct its own assessment. Given the enormous stress I was under in bringing Michael home, I would not have wanted to rely on my memory, let alone my medical skills, in devising Michael's health-care plan. A professional agency will involve you and your family when appropriate as it develops your plan of care. An initial telephone assessment will not do. A face-to-face evaluation is an industry-recognized standard.

Will the agency consult with your doctor or other professionals before developing the care plan? Such a discussion is important because it alerts the agency to any potential problems, whether health-related or drug-related, that might occur during the course of providing care. When you discuss the consultation, ask specifically that your doctor be called.

Does the agency assess your spouse's ability to perform the normal activities of daily living? I didn't want an agency that was going to treat Michael as a helpless and useless invalid.

On the other hand, my husband was a double amputee, so I wasn't about to hire any agency if its personnel considered it too much trouble to cook meals or facilitate his movement around the house.

Does the agency consider your home environment? Financial situation? Available social support? Our home health-care agency may have worked with hundreds of patients with diabetes but, as is the case with a good doctor, it treated individuals, not simply "textbook diseases."

Will you receive a written, detailed plan after assessment? How flexible is it? The plan should spell out the duties of all home health-care personnel, whether nurses, therapists, or aides. Even so, this does not mean that you have to settle only for those services listed on paper.

Let me give you an example. Our contract with the home health-care agency stipulated that their employees would cook meals for Michael. On occasion I asked the person who was cooking to make enough for me as well. At other times, I asked an aide to pick up pills at the pharmacy. I found that, in general, the agency's employees were more than happy to do anything that would make life easier for Michael and me.

If you are satisfied with the agency's answers at this point, ask about its supervision policies. Equally important, ask who provides the supervision and when that person is available. You should reject any agency that limits supervision of care-giving personnel to the telephone alone. If skilled nursing care is required, the nursing supervisor should periodically visit you. Use one hard and fast rule taken from Medicare standards: *If you need the services of a nurse, home health aide, or therapist, an in-home supervisory visit by a registered nurse at least once every two weeks is required.* At a minimum, the supervisor should be available during working hours to home-care personnel, you, and your family.

Of course, your spouse's health-care needs are not determined by the clock. Make sure you have a way of reaching a nurse in case of an emergency. Our agency operated a twenty-four-hour emergency answering service. Its nurses, supplied with beepers, could respond quickly to a crisis. This was equally true on evenings, weekends, and holidays.

Emergency or not, you need the peace of mind that comes with knowing you can reach someone for help. You may discover one day when you're about to leave for work that the morning nurse has not arrived. Nurses are human, too, and they will occasionally oversleep, wind up in traffic jams, and experience other delays, as do the rest of us. Always keep the agency's phone number, as well as the nurse's, at your fingertips.

Obtaining Sickroom Equipment

Michael and I were lucky. Our home health-care agency supplied us with all of the medical equipment we needed. You, however, might have to shop for many of these items on your own. If so, remember that the "Hospital Equipment and Supply" section of the yellow pages is only one source for obtaining what you need.

There are numerous other good sources for sickroom equipment. Dealers, hospitals, home health-care agencies, household retailers, and local pharmacies all sell or rent these wares. You have choices. Manufacturers print catalogs and hold trade shows in which they demonstrate the latest inventions for convalescing patients. Make friends with your local equipment dealer. He or she is generally happy to supply you with manufacturers' catalogs so you can see what is available in addition to what your local dealer has in stock. I was bombarded with catalogs once I let my interest be known.

Don't overlook possible sources of free loaner equipment. Patient and staff organizations such as the Visiting Nurses Association, the Heart Association, the American Cancer Society, the Veterans of Foreign Wars, the Muscular Dystrophy Association—and even some private organizations run by individuals—often lend equipment free of charge. Friends and relatives are other possible sources. They may have equipment they no longer need.

If you obtain sickroom equipment from a commercial source, *your most important consideration is good service.* A malfunctioning feeding pump or inoperative oxygen system could spell the difference between life and death. In *The Home Health Care Solution,* Janet Zhun Nassif recommends asking equipment providers the following specific questions:

- Is the provider Medicare certified?
- Will the dealer assist with inventory control?
- What happens if repairs are needed that cannot be done on the spot? (I was guaranteed replacement equipment within four hours.)
- If equipment malfunctions, will the dealer replace or loan other equipment at no extra charge?
- Does the dealership do its own repair and maintenance?
- Does the dealership offer seven-day, twenty-four-hour service?
- Does the dealership employ at least some service and professional staff on a full-time basis? What training do these employees receive?
- Does the dealership make in-home visits at no extra charge?
- Will the dealership train you and your family in proper equipment use and care?
- If you are purchasing used equipment, does the dealership provide spare parts?
- Does the equipment dealership maintain a list of contractors that widen doors or make space alterations?

Finally, *do not be afraid to bargain with the equipment dealer.* Ask for the manager or owner. Determine who has the authority to make a better deal. You might, for instance, suggest renting an item for the time being and then applying part of the rent to the purchase price if you later decide to buy it. Don't be intimidated by policy manuals. Remember that *everything is negotiable.* Policy manuals do not set hours and prices. Owners do.

Finding Short-Term and Long-Term Help

When our insurance policy no longer covered nursing services, I hired someone to come in and take care of Michael for several hours daily. *Knowing I was able to walk out of the house for those few hours every day was a major factor in helping me maintain my own psychological health.* It gave me a modicum of freedom and kept me in touch with my own needs.

Engaging short-term or long-term help on your own involves a considerable amount of work. As an employer, you will need to screen personnel, provide supervision, and complete paperwork for the IRS—at the same time that you balance family and job responsibilities. The built-in services of a home health-care agency—patient assessment, employee supervision, physician consultation, and so on— may be worth more to you than what you save by doing it all yourself.

Although you will find advertisements in the yellow pages and the employment sections of the newspaper, there are less risky ways of filling your needs. The personnel office at your hospital, the social-service staff at senior centers, an organization that serves people with your spouse's illness, a friend or family member, your clergyman—all may be able to provide the names of reliable employees. If you are looking for a nurse, you may want to contact the Visiting Nurses Association, which has links to many hospitals. Don't overlook senior citizens as possible employees, provided there is no heavy lifting involved. If there is a senior citizens' employment service in your community, it may be able to recommend just the person you're looking for. And don't rule out help that may be free; call hospitals to see if they can recommend volunteers.

What we are talking about here is "networking." In the business world it is generally used to find jobs or clients, and all it involves is letting people know what you are looking for. In this instance you're looking for qualified and reliable help to care for your spouse.

Good networking starts with the people who are most likely to be able to help you. I began by talking to the licensed practical nurses (L.P.N.) that the nursing agency had sent to care for Michael. I asked them if they knew anyone they'd recommend. Then I called the nursing service and asked if there was anyone they'd interviewed who didn't have the required professional degrees but whom they had liked. That led us to the woman we ended up hiring. She was the first and only person we interviewed. Michael and I both talked to her then checked her references. We had the gut feeling she was perfect for the job, and we were right.

The selection of a home health-care nurse or aide provides an excellent opportunity to involve your spouse and children in care-giving decisions. Whomever you select may be spending a significant amount of time in your home, so it is usual to include family members in the initial interviews. The reasoning is you may not be as objective on your own as you need to be.

Michael tried to delegate all hiring decisions to me, but I insisted he make the final choices. This gave him the opportunity to exercise considerable control over his environment and his quality of life, and I felt that was important.

Assuming that the employee provides credible references and that your family feels comfortable with him or her, your next step is to consider the particulars of your situation. *This is the time to speak up.* If you do not like smoking or require someone with a driver's license to run errands, say so. One of our night nurses smoked. Freezing cold or not, if she wanted a cigarette she had to go outside the house, and this was made quite clear to her before she took the job.

Make sure no aspects of your spouse's condition will pose problems for the potential employee. If your spouse is prone to temper tantrums, let the person know. If your spouse soils the sheets, needs to be lifted, cannot go to the bathroom unassisted, or has other difficulties, mention these things before you hire someone. Make a list of these problems so you won't overlook anything. This is highly important. It's a lot easier to weed out the wrong applicants before you engage someone than it is to hire the person you believe is ideal only to have him or her quit after the first day.

No matter whom you hire, be sure that you keep a backup list should that individual be unavailable for work. Keep in mind too that there is nothing wrong with hiring your relatives. We employed our children on occasion, and Michael loved the company.

Your method of phrasing requests is critical in getting the best service possible. Here are some key phrases I found helpful in purchasing home health-care services:

For the Equipment Dealer

- "I know this is short notice, but . . ."
- "Is there any possibility that . . . ?"
- "What are your normal hours of business? Is there any flexibility in that policy?"
- "Are you the manager? Is this your store?" (Your objective here is to get the best deal.)
- "Can we rent this for now and apply part of the rent to the purchase price if we decide to buy?"

For Short-Term and Long-Term Employees

- "That was a very creative and tasty meal."
- "Let's sit down today and figure out some new ideas for the cranky one."
- "My spouse really loves . . ."
- "If you get a chance today, could you . . . ?"
- "Can you help me understand that procedure?"
- "Tell me about your family/job goals/reasons for choosing this profession."

The more you get to know your equipment dealers and the people who are helping you in your home, the more likely they will offer help in an emergency. Because you have taken an interest in them and in their situation, they will be much more likely to take an interest in yours.

Coping Creatively with Health Care

We have talked at length about what others can do for your spouse. At this point, I'd like to offer a few tips from my own experience on things you can do yourself to make home care simpler and more cost-effective.

- Move an apartment-size refrigerator into the bathroom. Each morning check for juice, cold water, and other necessities.
- Place a thermos beside the bed. Contents stay cold all day.
- Place a scatter rug beside the bed to absorb spills.
- Make sure that the bedside table contains useful items like a telephone, clock, good reading lamp, notepad and pen, stationery, books, and magazines—and that a wastebasket is easily reachable.
- If your spouse is well enough to make it to the kitchen, rearrange the refrigerator so that commonly used items are within easy reach. I used a lazy Susan to make the back items more accessible.
- Attach a small, rolling TV table to the wheelchair so that food can be carried from one room to another.
- Place nonskid rugs by the kitchen sink and the tub.
- Install an intercom near the bed. Alternatively, a small dinner bell works well for summoning help (or company!).

Your needs will vary, but with a little creativity you can help your spouse live more pleasantly and independently. Start the creative process by thinking about what your spouse *can* do, and go from there. If he can lift himself, for example, then a trapeze and a smooth board will make parallel movement possible from bed to chair.

Don't forget the importance of a pleasant environment. There were times when Michael said, with great anguish, "You don't know what it's like to stare at these walls all day." When we redecorated our bedroom, I paid a particular amount of attention to the decor to the extent of putting in unusually attractive ceiling light fixtures so that Michael had something nice to look up at from his bed.

If the patient will no longer be sleeping in the master bedroom, choose a room that is logical for his or her needs. If quiet is a requirement, pick a room away from most family activity. If the person wants (or should be encouraged) to participate more in the daily action, choose a room more centrally located. Some caregivers put a bed in the living room or family room so that the sick person actually becomes the focal point of the family. Whichever room you choose, make it as comfortable, familiar, and cheerful as possible. Choose the pictures with care. Set out photographs of friends and family. Keep plants and pretty flower arrangements within sight.

The Coming-Home Checklist

You've contacted the home health-care agency, the home-health aide, and whatever equipment supplier you will be using. You've asked them all the right questions and gotten all the right answers. You're almost ready to bring your mate home—but not quite. There are still some important questions you need to ask *yourself.* How well have *you* prepared for the homecoming? How thoroughly have you prepared your home? The items below are what I consider the most important ones from my personal checklist. I offer them in the hope they will stimulate you to think of others that apply to your particular situation.

Have you:

- Checked for any physical obstacles or made any necessary space alterations? (Are wheelchair ramps in place? Have bathroom and kitchen doors been widened if necessary?)
- Arranged your home to guarantee your spouse maximum independence?
- Checked for safety hazards? (Loose wires, slippery floors, sliding scatter rugs, a water heater thermo-

stat set high enough to scald, and so on.)
- Called the pharmacist in advance for any necessary prescriptions?
- Made yourself a list of important telephone numbers in case of an emergency? This is also important for the use of home health-care employees.
- Made yourself a list of backup employees in case the person you hired is unavailable?
- Arranged for transportation to necessary services such as physical therapy or the doctor? If your mate has a problem that prevents full use of the legs, I highly recommend hand controls for his or her car. Even though Michael was a double amputee, he eventually was able to drive himself to the office and to dialysis. He could also avail himself of the services of drive-in banks, drive-in restaurants, drive-in dry cleaners, and the like—and gained a great feeling of independence in doing so.
- Placed a calendar near the telephone for quick reference?
- Let your children and close family members know in advance what they can do to help?

Plan in advance. Ask tough questions. Involve your family. Rely on creativity—yours and other people's. Follow these suggestions, and your spouse's homecoming can be the welcome relief you both have hoped for.

Bear in Mind:

Consider caring for your spouse at home as much as possible. The responsibility of caring for someone at home is stressful, but not nearly so stressful as having them in the hospital.

Carefully research home health-care agencies. Few of us would randomly select a doctor or a hospital, yet that is how many people select a home health-care team.

Remember that round-the-clock service does not necessarily indicate superior quality of care.

Do not be afraid to bargain. Everything is negotiable. Policy manuals do not set hours and prices—owners do.

Set aside time for yourself. Knowing I was able to walk out of the house for a few hours every day helped me maintain my own psychological health.

Recognize that there is nothing wrong with hiring your relatives.

14
Alternative Care Options

Sometimes as chronic illness progresses, there comes a point when, sadly, even the best care at home ceases to be care enough. Only a short time ago, options beyond home care were few. You could either admit an individual to a hospital for a brief stay with your doctor's consent or place the patient in a nursing home. Today, due to a combination of hospital cost-cutting measures, the rise in two-career couples, and the shortage of affordable nursing-home care, these options have been joined by additional choices designed to meet our changing needs.

Adult Day Care and Other Respites

If caring for a chronically ill person around the clock has left you emotionally and physically exhausted or is not possible due to job commitments, some form of respite care may be your answer. By providing health care for the dependent family member, respite care offers the caregiver just what it promises—a welcome period of relief. For some families it has helped postpone or even completely eliminate the necessity of a nursing home.

Hospitals, patient organizations, and social-service groups may offer respite services on either an in-home or extended-respite basis. The Alzheimer's Foundation, for example, sponsors a program that trains respite workers to watch a patient in the patient's home, giving the caregiver a break for all or part of the day. Some hospitals, including Veterans Administration facilities, offer extended respite services where the average stay is close to two weeks.

Perhaps the most popular respite service to emerge in recent years is the adult day-care center. Ideally, adult day care provides health and social services in a safe, comfortable setting to adults with physical or mental limitations. In addition to promoting health and independence, the programs offer activities and personal care to meet individual needs.

Adult day-care programs are often limited to persons who have particular illnesses, are over a certain age, or live in the immediate community. And adult day-care centers vary as much in their structure as in the patients they serve. They may be either private or public, profit or nonprofit. Some are located in senior citizens' centers, others in nursing homes, hospitals, churches, or buildings of their own.

An effective day-care program offers numerous advantages for the caregiver. It can improve the physical and mental well-being of the patient, making your care-giving tasks easier. You will also find it easier to care for your mate if you have a chance to rest or resume your normal activities. In addition, you might find that the break improves your relationship by lessening resentment engendered by lost independence, social activities, or simple exhaustion. If an illness progresses, adult day-care may allow you to continue home care longer than would otherwise be possible, thus minimizing costs and enhancing your spouse's quality of life.

A good way to start looking for an adult day-care center is by calling your local council on aging, a multipurpose senior center, the National Council on Aging, your local branch of the Visiting Nurses' Association, or your home health-care agency. *It is important to begin your search well before your situation necessitates respite care because adult day-care centers often have long waiting lists for admission.* In addition, it is much easier to make this important decision when you and your spouse are calm rather than under the pressure of a crisis.

Most adult day-care centers are small and are staffed by nurses, social workers, and activities directors. Frequently a center employs a specific individual, such as a social worker, to handle information and referrals. This doesn't mean you can't also arrange an appointment with the center's director if you desire. I recommend doing so. No matter whom you interview, it is important to state clearly your spouse's individual needs. Remember, you are not looking for a babysitting service but rather for a multiservice adult day-care program that will make a positive contribution to your husband or wife's quality of life—and to yours.

The National Council on Aging has prepared a consumer checklist of questions to aid you in your search for the right adult day-care facility. It can be obtained by writing to NCOA, CHOICES, 600 Maryland Avenue SW, West Wing 100, Washington, DC 20024.

Unfortunately, Medicare and private insurance companies do not pay for adult day-care. They may, however, finance certain medical and therapeutic services offered by adult day-care programs. In many states, the Medicaid program will pay the cost of such services for those persons with low enough income and few enough assets to qualify for care. Government funds may be available through programs such as the Older Americans Act or Supplemental Security Income to pay part of the basic fee. Since you will be paying for at least some portion of your spouse's adult day-care, you will need to determine what constitutes a reasonable fee. Costs vary from one community to another, so your best bet is to contact either your insurance company, the National Council on Aging, or the National Institute on Adult Day Care. Remember in estimating your costs that you can avail yourself of adult day care when it is convenient for *you*. You are not required to sign up for five-day weeks.

Choosing a Nursing Home

The idea that your life partner may need to be cared for in a nursing home can be both saddening and depressing. Many of us put off thinking about it until the pressure of making a decision is upon us. This is the wrong thing to do. Such crisis action can result in inferior care for your spouse and a lot of problems and trouble for you.

If your spouse has been diagnosed with a degenerative disease, shows warning signs of deterioration, or needs round-the-clock health care that you and your family, even with the aid of community services, are having difficulty providing, it is time to begin investigating the option of a nursing home. Because your spouse deserves special consideration in choosing a place to live, it is best to make this important decision when he or she is still alert and able to participate in it.

Preliminary sources of information on nursing homes are many: your local area agency on aging, senior citizens' centers, the United Way, the social services department at a major hospital, clergymen and workers with religiously affiliated social service agencies, your local branch of the Visiting Nurses Association, friends and relatives familiar with individual homes, and nursing-home residents whom you know personally. In addition, some communities have citizens groups that visit nursing homes and publish consumer information based on these visits. Your local chapter of the American Association of Retired Persons might be able to direct you to such a group.

Regardless of where you begin your search, ask yourself the same question you would in purchasing any medical service: "What kind of care will my spouse need?" Your doctor should be able to tell you what type of facility is

required and what special services or programs are necessary. The answer may be an acute care facility or simply a
place that's safe and comfortable to live in or something in
between. Bear in mind that your spouse's condition may
deteriorate at a later date. A setting that offers maximum
care can save you a troublesome move.

Unlike adult day-care centers, which are not licensed in
every state, all nursing homes should have current, permanent licenses. Eliminate any home with merely a provi-
sional license as well as any that has received an unfavor-
able annual state inspection. (You may obtain a nursing
home's inspection report through the nursing home om-
budsman in your state or area; your state agency that deals
with aging can put you in touch with him or her.) Eliminate as well any home located too far away from friends,
loved ones, or emergency medical facilities.

Once you've narrowed the field to this extent, find out if
a prospective nursing home has a vacancy and, if so, what
its admission qualifications are. If your spouse will be
placed on a waiting list, learn about the policy regarding it.
Is the list organized according to medical condition, date of
application, financial resources, or some other criterion?

As for admissions requirements, they will vary from
home to home. Some homes limit entrance to state residents. Others do not accept invalids. Still others reject
patients with serious mental disorders.

If you are pleased with what you've learned thus far
about a particular nursing home, schedule an appointment
with the director or with an administrator who is fully
informed about the operation. Tell him or her you would
like to meet with administrators and key personnel, such as
the Director of Nursing and the Director of Social Services. Arrange to watch a meal being prepared and served.
Taste the food. Ask to see as many different therapy
sessions and patient activities as possible.

As you tour the home, observe not only the physical
surroundings (rooms should be clean, well-lit, cheerful;

floors should be dry and free of clutter; hallways should have handrails, etc.), but also the employees and the patients. Do the patients interact well with the staff? Are they well-groomed? Talk with several patients. What do they think of the care they receive in the home?

Pay particular attention to the nursing home's medical and nursing services. If your spouse will depend on the house physician, make a point of meeting him or her. Ask what arrangements have been made for handling emergencies in the nursing home and for emergency transfers to the hospital. Visit with the nurses and ask them to explain the calling system by which residents can signal for help. Find out how drugs are safeguarded and who is authorized to administer them.

Once you have completed your tour of the facilities, it is time to discuss costs. Two sobering facts should convince you of the importance of this: as of this printing, the *average* yearly cost of a nursing home was in excess of $22,000! Neither regular private insurance policies nor Medicare cover long-term care. Medicare, in fact, covers only one hundred days in a nursing home.

Fully two-thirds of privately paying patients end up on Medicaid. This means they must first exhaust their resources until they reach Medicaid's eligibility level of no more than $1,800 in individual assets, excluding house, car, and home furnishings. Given this worrisome information, even if your spouse enters a nursing home as a privately paying patient, select a home that participates in both Medicare and Medicaid programs.

Whether you are financing nursing-home care with a long-term insurance policy, with a retirement or pension plan, or with public funds, you must take into account that the average basic monthly nursing-home charge does not include the "extras." Although the basic charge usually covers room and board, housekeeping services, recreation, and general nursing care, you will usually have to pay extra for such specialized diagnostic and personal services as dentistry, laboratory work, or beautician services.

If you shop competitively, you should be able to find a home that provides quality care at a reasonable price. Once you have found the best nursing home for your spouse, you will be asked to sign a contract. *Beware of any contract that requires you to sign away your real and personal property in exchange for care.* Do look for a contract that states in detail your costs, the services offered, and the legal obligations incurred by you and the nursing home. Rather than sift through pages of confusing legal terminology, *hire a lawyer to review the contract; the fee for this service is minimal compared to what you will pay for nursing-home care.* The American Bar Association Commission on the Legal Problems of the Elderly, the Health Advocacy Services section of the American Association of Retired Persons, or your local office of Legal Aid can supply you with the names of lawyers who will help you go over the contract before signing it. *Financing nursing-home care is a major commitment. Do not enter into it without securing the best advice available.*

Continuing Care Retirement Communities: The New Alternative

Because permanent nursing-home care exacts an extraordinary toll from chronically ill patients and their families, many older Americans have opted for an alternative to traditional nursing-home care that guarantees that they and their families will never be bankrupted by soaring medical expenses. The continuing care retirement community (CCRC), also known as a Life Care Community, is an innovative concept in health care.

Typically, residents pay an initial entrance fee plus a monthly charge for guaranteed housing and medical care. Residents usually live in independent dwelling units and sign a contract that guarantees occupancy but not ownership rights. If you decide after the move is made to a CCRC that the situation will not meet your needs, most facilities will refund a percentage of your entrance fee, figured on a sliding scale over a limited period of time.

A good CCRC provides security, independence, companionship, and health care. Prospective inhabitants purchase its services while still in reasonably good health, much as they would an insurance policy; of those who join the community, only one-quarter will ever need nursing care on a permanent basis. In return, the best life-care communities offer numerous amenities, including medical attention at the pull of a cord, transportation, apartment cleaning, group dining rooms or restaurants, doctor's offices, beauty salons, libraries, clubs, banks, and if needed, unlimited medical care at no extra charge in a nursing center on the premises. As in a hospital, communal facilities are connected by enclosed, weather-protected corridors.

The cost of all these services is quite high; therefore some CCRCs have converted certain services into options. Others have eliminated nursing care and entrance fees. Still others offer condominium units that the resident or the estate can later sell. Finally, some CCRCs have rented their units with the stipulation that they will help the residents find nursing homes or hospital care if their health deteriorates to the point where they must leave.

Not every community that designates itself a CCRC will offer all the services you need. Some centers require supplemental medical insurance to cover acute hospital care. Some exclude preexisting conditions from coverage. Others charge additionally for nursing services. Still others may maintain their own nursing homes and, although offering to refund an entrance fee and allow discontinuance of monthly payments if a resident must move there, will still charge substantially for nursing-home care.

Because CCRCs are a relatively new phenomenon, your biggest concern after deciding whether a community fulfills your needs is to assess its financial strength. You are taking a big risk if you select a new community, especially if the people behind it have no track record. Using the money from entrance fees to get started, developers frequently sell some contracts before building. Opening the doors too soon has been a leading cause of failure. Before making a financial commitment, ask for a written guarantee that ground will not be broken until at least half the contracts have been sold. Insist that the community's financial statements include plans for a reserve account for unforeseen costs. Ask these questions whether you are investigating a profit or not-for-profit facility. Even though a nonprofit group may have your best interests at heart, if that company goes bankrupt you will be affected. It should be noted, however, that nonprofit CCRCs are more lenient regarding occasional late payments of fees by their residents. The American Association of Homes for the Aged reports that it is rare for a contract to be terminated by a not-for-profit community because of inability to come up with monthly fees.

If you decide to sign a contract with a CCRC, hire a lawyer to review it and warn you of any provisions that could spell trouble in the future. To get more information about CCRCs, contact the American Association of Homes for the Aging, the American Association of Retired Persons, or the National Consumers' League. Other good sources include the office of aging in your area, your state department of health or insurance, and state and local consumer protection agencies.

The Hospice Option

Hospice is a concept of care, not a place or an institution. It is designed to serve the terminally ill. Unlike most medical institutions, a hospice does not serve a curative function. The members of a hospice team—which include health professionals, bereavement counselors, family members, and friends—provide emotional support to the dying individual.

Although most hospices in the United States involve caring for a patient in his or her home, hospices may also be based in hospitals or long-term care facilities. Regardless of a hospice's source, its goals remain the same: to provide a caring environment in which a terminally ill patient may die with dignity and to foster in the caregiver a lasting change in knowledge, attitude, and behavior regarding death. A hospice views death as a natural part of life. Norman Cousins, in his *Anatomy of an Illness*, explains why today's hospitals create a need for hospices:

> Death is not the ultimate tragedy of life. The ultimate tragedy is depersonalization—dying in an alien and sterile area, separated from the spiritual nourishment that comes from being able to reach out to a loving hand, separated from a desire to experience the things that make life worth living, separated from hope.

To learn about hospice programs in your area, we suggest you consult your hospital's office of continuing care, the National Association of Hospices, or even the yellow pages. If you have a friend, relative, or acquaintance who has participated in a hospice program, he or she may be your best source.

Not all states license hospices, and a state license is not sufficient in itself to guarantee the quality of services provided, so thoroughly investigate before becoming involved. At a minimum you will want to select a hospice that includes a pain-control program, counseling for the bereaved, pastoral care, and volunteers. Ask to speak with the medical director, and seek assurances that the program keeps detailed medical records.

The hospice's staff will help with insurance problems, wills, and funeral arrangements, as well as legal and financial matters pertaining to death. As for costs, few hospices will reject a prospective patient on the basis of inability to pay—a real benefit of the hospice option.

While the possibility that you may one day be unable to care for your mate in the home the two of you have shared together is not a pleasant thought, you have more alternatives to choose from today than at any previous time. Adult day-care, respite care, continuing care retirement communities, nursing homes, and hospice programs are all available to meet a full range of needs that home care cannot fill. With advance preparation and thoughtful selection, you should be able to find a program that meets your requirements and enhances the quality of life for both your spouse and you.

BEAR IN MIND:

Take advantage of alternative care options. Respite care offers the caregiver just what it promises—a welcome period of relief.

Investigate adult day-care choices. Adult day care may allow you to continue home care longer than would otherwise be possible, thus minimizing costs and enhancing your spouse's quality of life.

Remember, in estimating your costs, that you can avail yourself of adult day care when it is convenient for you.

Make the choice of a nursing home while your spouse is still alert and able to participate in the decision.

15
Rehabilitation, Support, and Counseling

A fter his first amputation, Michael began physical therapy to build his upper body strength. He was going to need it in order to walk on crutches while learning to use his new prosthesis. Although we did not realize it then, when he entered rehabilitative therapy Michael had become part of a dynamic new industry.

The combination of hospital cost-cutting measures that limit how long a patient stays and the growing public awareness that home care may be safer and more pleasant than hospital care has spawned a whole new field of outpatient and home rehabilitative services. Trying to sort out all the new options available and decide what's right for you isn't always an easy task. Your physician or surgeon can be of invaluable help here. In fact, it's most often the patient's doctor who specifies physical therapy. In twenty-two states, however, it is now possible for a patient or caregiver to engage a physical therapist without a doctor's prescription. And no doctor's order is required to set up an appointment with an occupational therapist.

The rehabilitative therapy industry is young, chronically understaffed, and still in the process of defining itself. It is generally agreed, however, that physical therapy, occupational therapy, and speech pathology form the new industry's core services.

Most people receive rehabilitative therapy outside the

home, but whether your husband or wife does rehabilitative work at home or elsewhere, the process of selecting a therapist is essentially the same. One thing that needs to be carefully checked is your insurance policy. Some companies will only pay if therapy is received in a hospital on an outpatient basis. Others, including Medicare, will cover therapy received at home if you are able to furnish a valid reason for doing it there.

Therapy can be administered in a number of settings, including rehabilitation hospitals (found in most larger cities), the outpatient clinic of your hospital, university clinics, and medical schools. Home health-care agencies often have physical or occupational therapists working for them. And more and more physical, occupational, and speech therapists are opening their own offices and running private practices much as physicians do.

The first rule in obtaining rehabilitative services is to start early. The time to ask questions is during your spouse's hospital stay, well before discharge. Many excellent resources are available for selecting a therapist. Your hospital discharge planner, the local branch of the Visiting Nurses Association, community-based home health-care agencies, elderly services agencies, patient and staff organizations, the American Physical Therapy Association, religious and social service organizations, support groups, your state department of rehabilitation, and the physical therapy department of your hospital can all help you with the selection process.

Whichever services will be required, ask your doctor or a discharge planner in your hospital's office of continuing care to begin therapy in the hospital if at all possible. Then keep the program going once your spouse arrives home. Continuity of care is critical to the rehabilitation process.

Choosing a Physical Therapist

Physical therapists concern themselves primarily with problems of mobility and strength. They work with you and your spouse in developing, explaining, demonstrating, and facilitating an exercise program aimed at strengthening muscular function and enhancing mobility. Bedridden patients, through their enforced inactivity, might breathe shallowly and consequently deprive their muscles of oxygen. They often develop bedsores and in some cases contract phlebitis. A physical therapist can help your spouse prevent as much damage as possible and move toward retaining a healthy, functional life-style.

Physical therapists can help alleviate problems associated with high blood pressure, weakened heart muscles, neurological inflammation, or painful joints and tendons. Many of the exercises prescribed will also help reduce stress. In addition, physical therapists can teach the safest ways to use equipment and to ambulate. If balance is a problem, your spouse can be taught how to fall safely, check for injuries, and get up off the floor.

You might want to think of the physical therapist as a negotiator. Before developing a rehabilitation plan, the therapist gathers from you, the doctor, and your hospital's office of continuing care information on the level of functioning anticipated upon discharge. Ideally, you then discuss what is to be accomplished from physical therapy sessions.

What qualities should you look for in a physical therapist? First, establish whether he or she is technically competent, which is not always as easy as it seems. Start by determining that a prospective therapist is licensed to practice in your state. If registered as well, that means he or she also possesses at least a bachelor's degree. That alone, however, does not attest to a therapist's competence. In many states a therapist can pass a qualifying exam, leave the field for several years, and achieve recertification simply by paying a registration fee. And because of the shortage of rehabilitation personnel, not all physical therapy agencies are headed by persons with physical therapy backgrounds. It pays to check carefully.

Insist that the person has specialized training in treating patients with your spouse's particular illness. An understanding of its ups and downs and complications helps establish a realistic program for the patient and a good relationship between patient and therapist.

Once you've ascertained that a prospective physical therapist is technically competent, the next step is to schedule a consultation in which you, your spouse, and the therapist discuss concrete program goals. Be open about your spouse's idiosyncracies. This is important because even though two patients may share the same diagnosis and demographic data, their differing personalities might make the same goals feasible for one but not the other.

Having set your goals, you must now disabuse yourselves of one misconception about physical therapy. As one rehabilitation expert warns, "There is no pill the therapist can give the patient to make him independent again." In other words, rehabilitation takes a lot of hard work—work that can only be done by the patient. But as Michael discovered, the rewards are well worth the effort.

As caregiver, you can play a vital part in motivating your spouse in this all-important area. The most effective way for you to do this is strictly an individual matter. It depends entirely on your personality and your mate's. The trick is in realizing what works for the two of you—and what doesn't. Sometimes it's the opposite of what works for someone else. Selma, whose husband had to learn to walk again after a paralyzing fall, pushed him to try a little more each day. When I tried a similar approach with Michael, I got no results. That's when I learned that often what succeeds may be the very opposite of what you've tried without success for so long. When I backed away from the daily Why Don't Yous and quit pestering him about it, Michael really began to make progress in rehabilitative therapy.

It did wonders for his self-esteem. Now when I came home from the office we had show-and-tell, where he demonstrated his progress. Finally the day came when he walked on crutches from the bedroom to the kitchen, the biggest and most wonderful show-and-tell of all.

In choosing a physical therapist, you cannot underestimate the importance of compatibility. Michael and his therapist got along famously. Michael related to Ron almost more like a visitor he'd invited to our home than as someone who had been hired to come in and work. Ideally, your spouse should be the captain of the therapy team. One of the downsides of being a caregiver is that your spouse can come to view you as an authority figure. You become like the doctor or the nurses, simply one more person issuing orders. A good physical therapist will encourage rather than order your spouse to do things.

It's important to be sensitive to the degree of help you can most effectively give in rehabilitation. One way to help determine this is to talk with the professionals you're depending on—your doctor, your physical therapist, your home health-care team. Get their advice on how far to get involved. Only then can you accurately determine what your role should be. If you find that your approach has a negative effect, back off. When I exercised to Jane Fonda tapes I suggested that Michael join in and do his arm exercises, but he was always much more enthusiastic about working with Ron than with me. Ron was a different person to talk to, someone else from whom he could solicit advice.

Choosing an Occupational Therapist

Many times during Michael's illness I found myself wishing that there was some kind of efficiency expert who would step in to help me with Michael's functional problems of day-to-day living. What I didn't realize was that there are such people had I only known where to look. They are called occupational therapists.

Is your spouse limited to the use of only one hand? An occupational therapist can demonstrate how to dress with minimal difficulty. Does your mate frequently knock over bowls or glasses, spilling their contents on the bed or the rug? An occupational therapist can recommend glasses or bowls with suction devices on the bottom. Is your partner eager to cook or resume other household duties? An occupational therapist can observe his or her activities and then suggest the most efficient way of performing them within the limitations of the illness. Is your spouse climbing the walls because movie theaters and shopping malls are inaccessible? Our physical therapist showed Michael how to negotiate side steps in the movie theater; an occupational therapist could have shown him an easier way to drive there.

Choosing an occupational therapist is akin to choosing a physical therapist. Start by consulting the same sources— the Visiting Nurses Association, the rehabilitation department of your hospital, your home health-care agency, and so on. What is true of physical therapists in some states is true of occupational therapists in all states—you don't need a doctor's referral to engage one. Unlike physical therapists who must pass state licensing exams, occupational therapists are licensed nationally. Some states also require licensing, but any occupational therapist should be certified by the American Occupational Therapy Certification Board. This ensures that the therapist has completed at least a bachelor's degree, passed a national certification exam, and served an internship of at least six months with three months' training in both physical dysfunction and psychology.

Despite the differences in training, the occupational therapist shares many responsibilities with the physical therapist, and in many ways the activities of the two complement each other. Both are teachers. The physical therapist undertakes an assessment of the patient's physical needs and teaches the necessary exercise techniques, while the occupational therapist assesses the patient's daily needs and teaches the family how to better accommodate them.

Choosing a Speech Pathologist

Any illness or accident that causes trauma to the cerebrum

can affect the ability to speak. Strokes, brain tumors, and accidents are just a few causes of communication disorders. A speech pathologist is a specialist who diagnoses and treats individuals with this type of problem. Through an individually goal-oriented program, the therapist will work with the patient to restore functional communication ability to its maximum potential. The program may include the strengthening of weakened oral muscles, the retraining of brain patterns to form words and thoughts, patient and family counseling, and practical advice for everyday living. A doctor's order is not required for speech therapy except in hospitals or nursing homes or if your insurance policy will be covering the cost.

Speech pathologists work in a variety of settings. Although many are employed in elementary or secondary schools, others are employed in hospital outpatient clinics, rehabilitation hospitals, university speech clinics, community speech and hearing centers, and private practice. Your doctor, hospital discharge planner, the local chapter of the Visiting Nurses Association, county medical association offices, and the American Speech Language Hearing Association can also recommend speech pathologists in your area.

As is the case in selecting a physical or occupational therapist, your goal is to choose someone who is not only clinically competent but also familiar with your spouse's particular type of speech problem. For example, if your spouse has suffered a stroke, you will want to choose a speech pathologist who specializes in this area.

At a minimum the person you select should possess a Certificate of Clinical Competence (CCC) in speech therapy. This means that the therapist has completed a program of graduate study in speech language pathology or speech language and hearing science, passed the national certification exam, and completed at least nine months of clinical experience under the supervision of someone holding a Certificate of Clinical Competence. Do not worry if your spouse is assigned an intern who is still completing the nine-month clinical training program, because he or she will be supervised by an experienced speech pathologist.

Selecting a Therapist

Whether choosing a physical, occupational or speech therapist, the process is relatively the same:

1. Always check your insurance policy before initiating therapy. Ask not only what the policy covers, but *where* it covers these services—in the home, only in the hospital, and so on.
2. Make certain that the therapist is certified. *Physical therapists* are state licensed or registered. *Occupational therapists* must hold a license from the American Occupational Therapy Certification Board. *Speech therapists* must have a Certificate of Clinical Competence.
3. Check that the therapist is trained to handle your spouse's specific disability.
4. Select a therapist who together with your spouse will design a specially tailored program.
5. Select a therapist who will involve you and your family in the rehabilitation process.

One of the realities of any outpatient or home-care service is that at some point your insurance will no longer cover it. For this reason it's good to steer clear of any therapist who takes the attitude that he or she is the only person who can perform a particular service. It's up to you to see to it that your spouse's rehabilitative therapy can continue after the therapist is no longer directly involved. That means you must learn as much as you can about the process. By playing an active role, you are sending your spouse an important message—one that says you have confidence in his or her further progress.

Rehabilitation on Your Own

We have dealt mainly with rehabilitative activities that involve outside professionals. Much rehabilitation, however, need not involve any professional help at all. I am thinking here of Michael's three-wheeled vehicle and what a difference it made in his life. Easier to get about in than a wheelchair, it had the added advantage of putting him almost at eye level with people.

And use it he did. It gave him enormous freedom of a kind he feared he had lost forever. On his "tricycle" he could go almost anywhere—even down from the house to the boat dock and onto his boat. With this newfound mobility he was able to spend many happy hours out on the water with his fishing rod and have daily entertainment feeding the ducks that soon learned to regard him as their own personal source of food.

A lot of rehabilitation has to do with ingenuity. We had a carpenter build a platform over the floor of the car so that Michael could get his wheelchair out without having to lift it over the hump of the drive train. However you approach it, rehabilitation means getting back to normal or at least making your New Normal as much like the old one as you can.

Support Groups

Occupational and physical therapists assist in your spouse's rehabilitation, but where can *you* go for much-needed rehabilitation? No matter how many medical professionals you bring into your house, you will still shoulder the major burden of care. Recent figures published by the Government Accounting Office indicate that families, friends, and neighbors provide close to 90 percent of all care for chronically ill patients. The demands on the caregiver's time and energy frequently result in fatigue, stress, loss of social and economic opportunities—and sometimes family breakdown.

Virtually every medical professional with whom we spoke recommended support groups. Why, then, had so few of the caregivers we interviewed made use of them?

Caregivers' reasons for shunning support groups are numerous. Some appear valid. After all, who wants to commute miles to a hospital during the day only to return again at night for a meeting?

Joan, wife of a cancer patient, typifies many who do not attend support group meetings:

> One, you don't think you need them; two, you don't have time; and three, you don't know who to contact, so you don't even know how to start it.

Rose, an elderly woman whose husband has had several strokes, reacted with anger when the local hospital asked her to attend a meeting:

> Learn about strokes? I told them I didn't want to know any more about them. I think I've already read every book in the library. And, my gosh, you have to get somebody to stay at home while you go to those things!

Had Rose attended just one meeting, she might have learned how to find a sitter for her husband. Though she had spent nineteen years as a virtual prisoner in her own home, the investment of a few hours might have changed her life.

Many caregivers thought that listening to other people's stories would be depressing. But those who participated found comfort in knowing they were not alone. Ben, whose wife is a lupus patient, expressed it this way:

> It always seems to be such a relief to a lupus patient to find out that someone else has it and is able to deal with it. Going to the support group meetings, where

they can compare notes with each other, is very helpful.

Beth suffers from a severe, sometimes life-threatening allergic condition known as Ecological Illness (EI). Her initial reaction to the idea of a support group was not enthusiastic. "I'd spent enough time taking care of my illness as it was," she objected. "I simply didn't want to spend any more." Then she wrote a magazine article about her illness and was swamped by thirty-five phone calls in a week. Others who had her rare condition were desperate to share information. One of them started a support group for EI sufferers which Beth allowed herself to be talked into attending, and she's been a member of the group ever since:

> It's the most helpful thing I've ever done, as far as living with my allergies is concerned. Now I have more than a hundred people I can go to for information about how to cope with my illness, people who have been through it and dealt with the very same problems I have. Plus, I get the satisfaction of helping other people with their problems.

Some people shun support groups because they are uncomfortable with the idea of appearing helpless. If you find yourself thinking along these lines, remember that everyone in your situation has experienced these feelings. You don't have to go to a meeting to unload or listen to others unload if that is not what you want. If what you need is good information on caring for your spouse and an understanding group of people who have learned how to confront problems similar to yours, support groups are excellent places to go.

Finding the Best Group for You

Before scouting potential support groups, it's a good idea to ask yourself what you hope to get out of such a group. Setting goals and knowing what you hope to accomplish will help you decide which group is best for you. Do you want practical advice on treating and financing your spouse's illness? Do you need people whose situations are similar to yours, with whom you can share experiences and compare notes? Or do you want someone with whom to discuss in private your intimate feelings?

Begin your search with your doctor. Physicians, particularly specialists, are frequently in touch with local support groups that deal with the illnesses they treat, and many make a practice of recommending such groups to their patients. Begin gathering information while your spouse is still in the hospital. Hospitals employ social workers who specialize in both the medical and emotional components of illness, so they are often aware of the wide range of services available in the community. Another excellent source of information is the department of medical social work in any reasonably sized community hospital.

Hospitals frequently operate their own support groups. One hospital in Baltimore offered an eight-session course in caring for individuals who are elderly and frail. Group participants learned how to manage stress, how to lift and bathe patients, how to survey resources in the community (i.e., day-care centers, respite care, and transportation), and were given a host of other practical tips.

If you live in a community that has a medical school, you can contact the department that deals with your spouse's particular illness. If it is cancer, for example, you would call the oncology department and ask for referrals.

Large employers are another source for finding help. Several companies today maintain employee assistance programs. They have on-staff personnel or a contract with an outside agency to assist employees in coping with personal problems. One of the responsibilities of the employee assistance counselor is to gather information about available resources in the community.

Patient and staff organizations are another good source

of information. Some organizations, such as the Alzheimer's Foundation, operate their own education and support groups. Others cooperate with hospitals in education programs. The American Cancer Society offers a five-week, education program entitled "Living With Cancer," administered by nurses and social workers within the individual hospitals. The Diabetes Association encourages hospitals to hire what it calls "diabetes educators."

Religious and charitable organizations offer still another source of support services. The Jewish Family and Children's Service in Baltimore, for example, sponsors a support group for caregivers of chronically ill patients. Its social workers are also available to provide clients with counseling and to help them locate other services.

If you simply want information on how to obtain support services, the public relations office of organizations that deal with particular illnesses, such as the American Cancer Society or the Arthritis Foundation, can usually comply with your request. Even pharmaceutical companies are getting into the picture. Johnson & Johnson, in conjunction with the National Council on Aging (NCOA), has published a series of eight booklets with down-to-earth information on community resources, Medicare, Medicaid, legal and financial planning, home safety, housing, health professionals and paraprofessionals, and even care-giving tips for a relative who is far away. NCOA itself has published a "Guide for Caregiver Support Groups." The American Association of Retired Persons has a guide entitled "Your Home and Alternative Care Facilities." It also provides care-giving tips on audiocassettes.

If your search fails to turn up a support group that meets your needs, you might consider starting one yourself. It's really not that difficult. Beth's friend who started the support group for persons with Ecological Illness began by running an ad in the personals section of a local newspaper. A dozen people showed up for the first meeting, and double that number for the second. The group met one Saturday afternoon a month in the social hall of a suburban church, affiliated itself with a national EI support group, persuaded local and regional physicians and other health professionals who dealt with the problem to be guest speakers free of charge, and advertised the meetings for free in the community service columns of the newspapers. In two years the membership list grew to 250, with an active membership of fifty-plus.

Professional Counseling

At some point during your spouse's illness, individual counseling might offer more promise than support groups. Unfortunately, many people attach a stigma to this type of assistance, not realizing that psychiatrists and psychologists deal as much with "normal" people as with the mentally ill. Clinical psychologist Nancy Coniaris explains why caregivers sometimes are in need of professional help:

> When a very difficult, traumatic, and chronically wearing event enters your life—like your spouse develops cancer—it tends to strain you on the parts of yourself that are not so stalwart to begin with. You can get worn down and done in by things so that you end up not functioning as well as you might if life had been more problem-free.
>
> People frequently won't give themselves credit for being worn down for perfectly legitimate reasons. That kind of thing is difficult for a support group to get a grip on and work with. If the briefer kinds of services don't seem to be an enormous amount of help, people should be encouraged to see a more specialized person, like a psychiatrist. They're cheating themselves if they don't.

Dr. Coniaris offers the following advice:

> If you're feeling like the amount of difficulty you're having is puzzling and troubling, or that other people around you are complaining and thinking that there's

something the matter with you or the manner in which you're handling things, then that's a good time to get it checked out. A sophisticated person can help assess whether what you're struggling with is par for the course for the situation you're in.

How do you go about finding the right psychiatrist or psychologist for you? The average, reasonable person underestimates his or her ability to size up whether a therapist has any sense or not, even though the process is essentially the same as in choosing a doctor (see Chapter 12). Ask around for referrals and then begin interviewing, initially on the telephone. Any therapists who are competent will tell you a little about their approach. If they don't do that, you can eliminate them. The next thing is to go talk to them. Ask where they've trained, how long they've been working and how much they've done in this area. The good ones will take a minute to orient you. If not, or if they don't make sense to you, you're probably dealing with somebody who is not pleasant or who is incompetent. Watch out for people who are too sharp on the advertising, because there are a lot of therapists who are high on marketing and low on talent.

Rehabilitation presents a unique challenge. More so than when dealing with the hospital or securing home health-care nurses and equipment, successful rehabilitation demands that you and your spouse assume the ultimate responsibility for improving his or her health. Physical therapy works only if the exercises are willingly performed. Occupational therapy succeeds only if a person is committed to resuming the normal activities of daily life. Support groups are beneficial only if approached with a positive attitude. Psychotherapists can be of help only if you or your spouse is willing to make a serious effort to address difficult issues.

The sense of achievement you and your spouse can experience when you do these things for yourself is enormous. No nurse or pill in the world could have made

Michael feel any better than he did when he made up his mind to learn to walk from the bedroom to the kitchen on crutches and an artificial leg—and did it. It could not have happened any other way.

BEAR IN MIND:

Make sure your spouse is the captain of the therapy team.

Use your imagination. Much rehabilitation doesn't need to involve a professional at all; a lot of it has to do with ingenuity.

Realize that you must also have sources of rehabilitation for yourself. The demands on the caregiver's time and energy frequently result in fatigue, stress, loss of social and economic opportunities—and sometimes in family breakdown.

Check out support groups. Virtually every medical professional with whom we spoke recommended support groups.

Consider starting a support group yourself if your search fails to turn up one that meets your needs.

16
Determining Costs

W hen serious illness strikes your family, it is not uncommon to feel that you're at the mercy of just about everyone. Doctors, insurance agents, pharmacists, and even the clerks in the Social Security office can assume almost mythical stature when they have the power to deny your needs. Sometimes it can seem as if your entire existence is spent fighting for what is rightfully yours. Never mind that your mate is seriously ill. Never mind that you can justify and document every expense. You are up against an army of individuals trained in the art of saying no.

Against these obstacles, too many caregivers and their chronically ill spouses, whether out of fear, embarrassment, ignorance, or sheer exhaustion, fail to claim resources that are rightfully theirs. In the battle for benefits it is unfortunate but true that fairness takes a backseat to perseverance. It is up to you to persevere, to make it more difficult—and we would hope impossible—for those you depend on to say no.

How do you get from no to yes? How do you stay afloat in the face of staggering medical bills?

Maximize Your Resources

When I began this book, there were two points I wanted to

make above all: first, that you have options, even in the most trying situations; second, that it is up to you to maximize your resources.

In order to make the best use of the resources available, you have to determine what they are. Insurance policies, pension plans, and government entitlement programs are all resources. So are lawyers, financial planners, advocacy groups, and other caregivers who are or have ever been in your shoes. Take into account your insurance policy, salary, savings, Medicare, Medicaid, and disability benefits—the obvious things. But don't stop there. You've still got a long way to go.

Have you ever known a child who badly wants to buy something? It is amazing how creative he becomes. All of a sudden he remembers your past promise to pay him for a job. He remembers every ice-cream cone that was never consumed and every ball game that was never attended. He tries to exchange future Christmas or birthday presents for an immediate advance. There are lessons for us all in this child's tenacity and singleness of purpose. He expects a chorus of "no," but is willing to put up a fight anyway, and more often than not he will get his way. If you persevere, you too may get the "yes" you're going after. *If you dig deeply enough, you might find previously unconsidered sources of income or unknown savings.*

Have you checked to see whether telephone and utility deposits were refunded once you demonstrated that your credit record was satisfactory? Sometimes those deposits sit for years without earning you any interest. Have you checked to see whether your spouse has exhausted all of his or her sick days? That's another possible undiscovered resource. Have you called your government office of social services to find out if you qualify for assistance? Governmental assistance does not begin and end with Medicare, Medicaid, and Social Security. Have you attempted to negotiate the price of medications or diagnostic services with your physician or pharmacist? Have you explored ways you or your spouse might be able to earn money at home? If immediate cash is a problem, have you considered a home equity loan? Perhaps it's time for the two of you to sit down together and brainstorm for a list of resources, money-saving tips, and money-earning possibilities that apply to your situation.

Get the Most out of Your Insurance

Familiarize yourself with your insurance policy. Irene, who has cared for her diabetic husband for years, expresses the frustration of many care-giving spouses who learned "on the job" that medical necessity, in and of itself, does not guarantee coverage:

> I wish so much that doctors would sit down and say, "This is the situation and that is what it is going to cost." But instead they say, "Go have this transplant. Medicare pays for it." Well, that's just not true. Maybe Medicare pays for the operation, but it doesn't pay for the years of care and medication.

Imagine Irene's predicament when her husband's Medicare benefits ended only three years after he first became ill and he was left without coverage of any kind until he qualified for disability a year later.

Rose, a seventy-year-old woman who has been a caregiver for the past nineteen years, found out the hard way that insurance or disability payments go to those who fight rather than those who need them. The absurdity of the system hit home when, after numerous accidents, she purchased a trapeze to help get her 200-pound, stroke-disabled husband in and out of bed. Arguing that on the actual day of purchase he had not needed the trapeze, Medicare refused to pay. "Why would I buy a trapeze for a small apartment if I didn't need it?" Rose bellowed.

Rose had also been pushed aside when she applied for Social Security benefits on behalf of her husband. "I found out later that they always say no and that you fight it," she said, "but I'm not that type. If they say no, I figure that's what they mean."

Had Rose only known what you know now! No doesn't always mean no. If you know your rights under your policy, you can turn many a no into a yes.

In the deluge of worries brought about by chronic illness, nothing is more shocking than to have your umbrella of insurance yanked away without warning. This happened to Jack:

> One year Shelly was in the hospital thirteen times, and each time she stayed anywhere from four to eight days. She was sick so much that the company I worked for had its medical insurance cancelled. My boss got a new insurance policy with someone else, but of course they charged him a lot of money. He actually held that against me, because he had to pay much more. For a long time he wouldn't give me a raise.

If you find the wording in your policy confusing enough to make you wish fervently for a translator, rest assured that help is available. Such people do exist. AARP advises calling your state or county agency that deals with the aging, a good source of referrals for someone who can help you interpret the "insurance-ese."

Once you have reviewed the policy and determined that you do qualify for benefits, you still cannot assume that the insurance company will automatically pay all of your bills. Most only pay a fixed percentage of what is deemed the "reasonable and customary cost" of a given procedure in your geographical area. If your doctor or hospital charges more than that, the extra expense comes out of your pocket.

If you carry private insurance, call your agent and find out the reasonable and customary rate in your area for any procedure that your spouse requires. If the going rate is $500 and your doctor charges $1,000, you are going to end up paying $500. It seems fairly obvious that you should ask your doctor about the fee before accepting the service, but many people, usually out of embarrassment, refrain from doing so. Not unlike a bereaved family member who is easily pressured into buying an expensive funeral package, too many patients and caregivers fear that questions about cost will indicate stinginess on their part.

You may find yourself thinking, "How can I be cheap over something as important as my spouse's health?" If so, then perhaps it is time to say to yourself, "Of course I love my spouse, but I need to see to it that we don't burden ourselves any more than we have to." Remember, shopping for medical care is just good common sense.

If you qualify for Medicare, you can determine what constitutes a reasonable charge by consulting your local Medicare carrier. As is the case with private insurance, a charge is reasonable if it falls within the range that is customary in your area. Any charge above this will result in more out-of-pocket expenses to you.

One way to limit medical expenses is to choose physicians and medical professionals who accept assignment. This means that the doctor or supplier agrees to charge only the price allowed by Medicare for covered services and supplies and to handle all paperwork. Your local Social Security office can supply you with a directory published by Medicare carriers that will give you the names of physicians in your area who accept assignment and the percentage of cases in which they do so. Even if your doctor is not listed, it never hurts to inquire whether he or she will make an exception in your case.

Since Medicare regulations change frequently, you should know what is covered at any given time. The U.S. Department of Health and Human Services publishes a free pamphlet entitled "Your Medicare Handbook," which can be obtained from any Social Security office. It gives detailed, up-to-date explanations of the Medicare program and its two separate components, hospital insurance and physician insurance.

Bear in mind that Medicare is not a comprehensive health program. Nonetheless, it is the primary insurer for older adults, many of whom at some point exhaust its benefits. This is often the time when chronically ill patients apply for disability benefits. If you do not have private disability insurance, there are other disability benefit programs for which you might qualify. These include, but are not limited to, a State Worker's Compensation Program, Veterans Administration pension disability benefits, Civil Service disability benefits if you are a government worker, Black Lung benefits, and State Vocational Rehabilitation benefits. The Cash Sickness programs of California, Hawaii, New Jersey, New York, Rhode Island, and Puerto Rico provide income replacement to residents disabled because of nonoccupational injury or illness.

Cut Doctor, Hospital, and Lab Costs

There are a number of ways you can cut down on medical expenses by working with the health professionals who are caring for your spouse. We've already discussed selecting doctors who accept assignment and asking them what a procedure will cost. It is equally important to determine which tests and procedures are necessary, particularly if your spouse is entering the hospital. Duplication of blood tests, x-rays, and other diagnostic procedures is not only unnecessary but costly. *Keep a master list of all diagnostic tests and procedures performed,* with the dates they were done and the names of physicians who ordered them. This is particularly useful if your spouse is under the care of several different specialists, as is often the case with chronic illness. (See Chapter 12 for more about assessing tests and procedures.)

Another way of cutting lab costs is to arrange to be billed through your doctor rather than directly, because many laboratories charge a physician less than they do an individual patient. If, for instance, your husband or wife requires daily or weekly blood samples over an extended period of time, the savings to you can be considerable. Discuss this possibility with your doctor.

When surgery is recommended, ask for a second opinion. Medicare, your county medical society, or even your own doctor can supply you with the names of board-certified physicians to contact. The majority of private insurance companies, as well as Medicare, will cover you for second surgical opinions. Medicare will even cover you for a third if the first two do not concur. Although you might feel embarrassed by making such a request, insist that your doctor send all pertinent laboratory test results and medical files to the second physician to ensure that the latter has all the information needed. (See Chapter 12 for more information on the ins and outs of getting a second opinion.)

If your spouse must be hospitalized, there are things you can do to hold down costs. Did you know, for example, that teaching and for-profit hospitals are normally more expensive than their not-for-profit counterparts? To make sure you are not paying more than you must, try calling the business offices of nearby hospitals where your physician practices and check the prices of rooms and of the procedures you require. If the quality of care is comparable, choose the least expensive. If the procedure to be performed is not major, confer with the doctor to see if it can be done on an outpatient basis.

When you do check into a hospital, try to do so on a weekday. The earlier in the week the better. Most hospitals reduce their staffs on weekends and delay diagnostic tests until the following Monday, meaning that you can end up paying for an expensive "weekend hotel visit."

Just as there is no point in entering the hospital too early, there is no point in staying any longer than necessary. Let the physician know that you want your husband or wife to return home as soon as possible. Although hospitals routinely discharge patients earlier than they used to, some prompting on your part is still in order. If home health care is an option, why continue to pay for more costly hospitalization?

As with any major purchase, examine your hospital bill with a careful eye to make sure you haven't been charged for services not received. Bring any such matters to the billing office's attention as soon as possible, while all the details are still fresh in your mind.

Reduce Drug Costs

Prescription drugs for someone who is chronically ill often take a bigger bite out of a health-care budget than anticipated. One of the most effective ways to reduce such costs is to ask your physician to write prescriptions for generic drugs. The term *generic* refers to the chemical compound itself as opposed to the competing commercial name under which a drug might be sold. Generic drugs are every bit as safe as their brand name counterparts but sometimes cost only half the price. Even if you forget to ask your physician for a generic prescription, your pharmacist might still be able to make the substitution on request.

Another way to cut drug expenditures is to bargain for the cost of your medication much the same way we discussed bargaining for the cost of home health-care equipment in Chapter 13. Katy, an asthma patient whose prescription drug bills typically run from $300 to $400 a month, reports visiting a number of pharmacies and soliciting bids for her business. Huge differences in price can exist even between drugstores within the same neighborhood. The savings to you can add up to thousands of dollars over the course of a long-term illness.

Physicians are regularly bombarded with samples from pharmaceutical companies. If you ask your doctor for some of these, you'll not only save money initially but you can also find out whether a certain medication is effective before you invest in a large supply. Once you have determined a drug's effectiveness, you can save money by purchasing as large a quantity as will remain fresh at the rate you use it. Since the price of a prescription equals the cost of the medicine plus the pharmacist's dispensing fee each time the order is filled, buying in quantity will save you money.

Manage Your Money

It is just as important to manage wisely the money you have as it is to avoid spending unnecessary sums on medical care. Other bills don't disappear just because medical bills take center stage.

One sound resource many people ignore is the service of a financial planner. You don't have to be a millionaire to need or pay for sound financial advice. A financial planner can help you better utilize and maximize the resources you have. For example, he or she might point out important tax deductions or higher rates of return on your savings. A good financial advisor will give you a comprehensive, written plan to improve your present financial situation. He or she will identify problems while consulting with your banker, broker, insurance agent, or any other professional who handles your money. A good planner will also keep you abreast of any major changes in your financial situation or of laws that will affect your money. It is part of a financial planner's job to stay up-to-date on monetary matters.

For help in reviewing your assets and making a sound financial plan, the International Association for Financial Planning, headquartered in Atlanta, is a good place to start. A simple phone call can provide you with a list of registered members—all of whom meet its tough standards—in any city in the country, and with a booklet explaining how to select a financial planner and how the fee structure works.

The Institute of Certified Financial Planners, located in Denver, is another good source. It works closely with the College for Financial Planning, which conducts certification examinations and sponsors continuing education programs for financial planners in addition to maintaining a speakers' bureau and acting as a referral source.

Financial advisors generally charge either a flat or an hourly fee, a commission, or a combination of the two. As of this writing, hourly fees range from $50 to $150 and flat fees from $500 to $5,000. Most true financial planners expect to earn a client at least twice their fee in tax savings. If you are a novice, steer clear of planners who work on commission, as their advice could be consciously or unconsciously biased toward the programs or services they are selling. If your resources are modest, be open about this when seeking a financial consultant. Some advisors specialize in serving such clients; those who don't can probably guide you to someone who does.

That an individual is a lawyer, insurance agent, or accountant is not sufficient in itself to guarantee competency as a financial planner. Talk to a few planners. Ask them about their professional backgrounds, the length of time they've spent in the business, and the number of clients they have served. Ask for references. Determine whether they are registered with the Securities and Exchange Commission, which makes them subject to tighter controls.

You'll want to bring to the meeting your bank account, stock, insurance, and tax information. The better organized *you* are, the more time you'll save—and time is money if you are being charged by the hour. Any good planner will ask questions about you and not spend most of your appointment time proposing specific plans or exotic tax shelters. If you are pressured to delegate or abdicate your financial responsibilities or even to hand over some of your assets, walk out the door and don't look back.

If Possible, Work at Home

I heard an inspiring story about a telephone repairman whose wife was confined to a wheelchair. By purchasing an old switchboard for $200, he helped her create an

answering service that eased their debt burden and re-
stored her self-esteem.

Earning money at home often requires a great deal of
creativity and ingenuity. Here is an area where brainstorming and networking with as many people as possible can
really pay off. Start by telling everyone you know that you
and your spouse are looking for ways to earn money. Don't
neglect the services of your state department of vocational
rehabilitation, where you can get testing and counseling
that might help you choose a particular area to pursue.
Programs and services of the U.S. Small Business Association are also worth investigating.

The advent of the home computer has been a particular
boon to cottage industries. If you do not own a personal
computer and are not computer literate, you might want to
thumb through several computer magazines, pay a visit to
a computer store, or take advantage of computer literacy
classes offered as night adult education courses at many
universities. If you live in a reasonable-size city, watch for
free introductory workshops periodically offered by manufacturers such as IBM or Apple. Watch the newspaper for
ads, or contact your local computer store for information.

Unfortunately for those who want to start a business at
home, there is no shortage of unscrupulous operators out
there waiting to take advantage of you, particularly if you
are desperately strapped for funds. These individuals offer
to do what your insurance policy, savings pension, and
traditional sources of income won't—pay all your bills and
help you get rich to boot. If an offer of an investment
opportunity or at-home employment seems too good to be
true, it probably is. Even the most sensible people sometimes lose their heads when confronted with the emotional
strain and financial drain of a chronic illness. This is what
leads Rose, a well-educated librarian, to lament after years
of caring for her husband, "I know it's stupid, but I just
keep praying that some day I'll win the *Reader's Digest*
sweepstakes. I don't see any other way out of my dilemma."

Most work-at-home scams involve jobs stuffing envelopes or assembling small items. If an ad promises unrealistically high profits, guarantees huge markets and demand for your work, insists that no experience is necessary, uses personal testimonials without identification, or requires you to buy a starter kit or pay an initial fee to find out what is involved, it is most likely a scam. You will be better off seeking employment through your own networking efforts.

This is not the time in your life to risk gambling away your dwindling resources, so if you choose to earn money through investment opportunities, get recommendations from a reputable bank or brokerage firm. Be wary of investment opportunities advertised in newspapers or magazines; the happy investors appearing in the ads may be none other than those same individuals who are trying to make off with your money. Before you put your cash on the line, you might want to send for "Before You Say Yes: 15 Questions to Turn Off an Investment Swindler," available free of charge from the M. B. Woods Consumer Information Center, Pueblo, Colorado 81009. Specify pamphlet #570-R when requesting it.

Shopping for bargains, determining the best purchases, making sound investments, and earning money are always difficult. When you are under the stress of caring for a chronically ill person, they become all the more difficult. But you are not powerless. By educating yourself about the options available, you can make life more pleasant—and more secure—for yourself, your spouse, and your dependents.

BEAR IN MIND:

Don't be shy about filing for eligible payments. Too many people, whether out of fear, embarrassment, ignorance, or sheer exhaustion, fail to claim resources that are rightfully theirs.

Make a complete list of your assets. If you dig deeply enough, you might find previously unconsidered sources of income or unknown savings.

In the deluge of worries brought about by chronic illness, don't forget to check about your insurance. Nothing is more shocking than to have your umbrella of insurance yanked away without warning.

Comparison shop for prices of medications. *Huge differences in price can exist even between drugstores within the same neighborhood.*

Seek professional help in meeting expenses. *One sound resource many people ignore is the service of a financial planner.*

17
When the Illness
Is Terminal

If the doctors have done all they can and have informed you that your husband or wife has only limited time left, the two of you face a long journey. The first part of it can be made together. You can begin to say good-bye, both to each other and to life as it has been.

Then the road comes to a fork, and your spouse heads off into uncharted territory where he or she must come to terms with the unknown of death. Many dying individuals find this road easier if they are allowed to tie up any loose ends and take part in planning the ceremony of passing. Kathy Newman, a nurse who works with dying patients, explains:

> The people who can talk about their impending death have a peace and a serenity in the acceptance. They get so much out of the last part of their lives, and so do the family members who are able to talk and to be there and to tell each other how they feel. I look at it as almost a gift. We all know we are going to die, but these people have been given a certain amount of time and you would be amazed at how many of them have a lot of things they want to wrap up.

Your spouse is busy planning an ending. You, on the other hand, must begin to plan a future that doesn't include the one person you would most like to share it with. This crushing emotional burden is quite enough to cope with, but heaped on top of it await countless legal, financial, and personal decisions.

It is possible to work your way through a considerable number of these before the pain of loss confuses the issues. By taking certain legal and practical steps in advance, you can eliminate many of the complications that arise when a member of a family dies. In today's world these issues should be discussed by every married couple even when no illness is present. You are not doing your spouse a favor by sparing him or her the details of the family finances. Both partners in a marriage should get acquainted with the running of the household, what one friend of mine not-so-jokingly calls "widow training."

Legal Matters

The legal steps that you and your spouse can take to protect your assets often seem complicated to the layperson. I am going to touch on only a few of the basic arrangements. Since they vary so much from state to state and because I am not an attorney, I urge you to seek out sound legal advice—and to avoid do-it-yourself books that can lead you into decisions that will cost far more than an hour or two with an attorney would.

Encourage your terminally ill spouse to give someone he or she trusts—very likely you—*power of attorney* to make legal and other decisions. In many states, giving a spouse or a third party a power of attorney over one's affairs requires that the giving person be mentally competent to make that decision, so it is something that should be considered and done sooner rather than later. Exactly what a particular power of attorney covers can be specified, meaning that the areas of responsibility can be as narrow or broad as desired.

Other legal designations, such as *guardianship, living trusts,* or *conservatorship of property or person,* are also available; your attorney can give the best advice on what suits your particular situation. I have devised my own arrangement. In my present state of good health and in my new circumstances, I have established a three-person committee that will conduct my affairs if I am ever mentally unable to do so myself. I have diversified the group by choosing one child, one lawyer, and one friend, so there will be no possibility of, say, three children ganging up on the others. The three people I have chosen must agree on everything.

A *will* specifies how a person's estate will be divided upon his or her death. It is astonishing how many people are unaware of the importance of having a will. "The law will leave everything to my spouse, which is how I want it anyway," goes the rationale, "so why go to the bother and expense of making out a document that will serve exactly the same function?" Not only is that an incorrect interpretation of the intestacy laws (in some states only half of the estate will go to a spouse—the rest goes directly to the children), but a will can encompass far more than who is going to get the house and the money. It gives maximum choice in deciding not only how property is to be divided but how children are to be provided for, who will assume guardianship of young children if both parents die at once, how much money will be left to charities, or how friends as well as family will be taken care of. A will can protect the estate from some types of liability and can specify payment methods for debts and taxes. It can give items of sentimental value to chosen individuals.

Perhaps most importantly of all from the caregiver's point of view is that the creation of a will might save on state inheritance or estate taxes by arranging to make the best use of credits and deductions, and it might also save on the cost and time for probate. *Probate*—the legal settling of an estate—is where any potential problems with family members are likely to surface. Disagreements can cause lengthy delays in disbursement of money and property, and can leave the estate in limbo for months—sometimes even years.

The process of probate begins by inventorying property

and monies that were owned by the deceased on the actual date of death. During those first critical weeks, *keep a record of every penny you spend and of all deposits you make and where they came from*, because many of those expenditures will be expenses of the estate.

If the patient executes a will or other legal document while critically ill, be certain to have several witnesses who later can attest to his or her mental competency. A casual discussion before signing—perhaps on current events, politics, or sports—should test his or her alertness and awareness. Also be aware that formal will execution requirements differ from state to state in terms of the number of witnesses required, the formalities of the actual execution ceremony, and so on. If the person's health later improves significantly, it may be advisable to reexecute the document to avoid the possibility that someone will otherwise contest it on the basis of mental incompetency.

The legal costs of preparing a proper will are quite small in comparison to what your costs might otherwise be. A few hundred dollars now can save thousands later. In order to learn more about how probate problems can be avoided and taxes minimized, I strongly urge you to get professional advice from your lawyer, accountant, or other advisors.

Business Matters

Several other steps can be taken to protect you and your family, and once again the need for them varies from state to state. In some states you might be wise to avoid probate where possible, while in others probate is simple and inexpensive. I can't cover all eventualities here, so I will touch upon just a few to help you become aware of some of the possibilities.

Property. Encourage your spouse to think about the eventual disbursal of property. If most assets are to be left to you, in some states the easiest way of ensuring this might be to put real estate, and possibly certain other assets, into joint ownership. Some states require that "right of survivorship" or similar language be used in order to protect a person's rights to that property upon the death of the spouse. I used to see the letters JTWROS on many legal documents, but until I became a widow I never knew what those little letters meant or how important they were in my state. *Joint Tenant with Right of Survivorship* means that upon the death of one co-owner, title to the entire property goes directly to the survivor. In some states simple joint ownership, particularly if between spouses, implies survivorship, while in others it must be specified.

Safe Deposit Boxes. If important papers are stored in a safe deposit box, put that box in both of your names so that you have immediate access to it. If you live in a state that has an estate or inheritance tax, you may be required to open the safe deposit box in the presence of bank officials and state tax authorities so that an inventory can be made. Some people think that a safe deposit box should be secretly emptied before the bank is informed of the death, but you should be aware that this can subject you to charges of tax fraud.

Bank Accounts. What happens to bank accounts is again subject to state law. A good way to ensure that you will have access to enough cash during the first days and weeks is to keep at least one account in both of your names. Michael and I had individual checking accounts, but we also had a joint account for household use and I continued to have access to this entire account upon his death.

Utilities. In some areas of the country it might be advisable to put all utilities under two names so the survivor does not have to pay new deposits and installation charges to have accounts transferred to the new name. To find out, check with your local companies. In my area this wasn't necessary, but I've heard horror stories to the contrary. I trary. I did not transfer utilities into my name until after Michael's death. I then created a note that said: "It is with sadness that I inform you that my husband passed away on [date]. Would you please change your records into my name." I included a copy with every bill I paid.

Credit Cards. Put the primary ones into both names so that the survivor won't be left without credit.

Important Papers. Wills, deeds, titles, and other important papers should be stored where the chance of accidental destruction is minimal. If you lock the originals in a safe deposit box, keep copies on file at home since bank access may be delayed. You might want to buy a fireproof box or safe and store everything at home, although even then you should keep a copy or two of the will someplace else, such as with your attorney. Some attorneys' offices have fire-proof safes for storing clients' documents, so you could leave originals in their safekeeping and keep copies at home.

Begin collecting documents now so that you don't have to do this during the hectic first days after the death when you're in a state of shock, friends and relatives are arriving, and you have the funeral to get through. The checklist in this chapter suggests specific items to accumulate. Keep copies of everything in one easily accessible location.

Living Will

Like many people, Michael feared he would become a "helpless vegetable"; he could not stand the thought of being kept alive once the quality of his life diminished below a point that was acceptable to him. One way around this would have been to make out a living will to ensure that no heroic measures would be taken once he was un-able to maintain basic physiological functions on his own.

It used to be that the medical profession went to any extreme to prolong life, but now that technology makes it possible to keep people alive for years, even when their quality of life is poor, what used to be a "right to live" issue is fast becoming a question of "the right to die." As often happens with transitions, much turmoil accompanies it, and each case that comes to court breaks new ground. Finding answers to these many moral, legal, and religious questions will become imperative with the aging of the enormous baby boom generation.

As Katy discovered, even physicians aren't of one accord when it comes to living wills:

> My doctor in Florida couldn't deal with it at all because I was only in my late twenties. I said, "Well, it's a reality. I've been on a respirator nine times, and I do not want to go to the extremes. When my time comes to die, I've dealt with dying and I don't want to have all this scientific whatever." You have a choice in that, and I think you should be allowed to choose. We do some pretty barbaric things in this day and age to prolong death, just because we can't deal with that particular subject.

Thirty-eight states now have living will statutes that enable individuals to specify exactly what should or shouldn't be done to keep them alive, although state laws vary over whether the provision of food and water is mandatory. Included in a living will can be the appointment of someone trusted to act as "proxy" once a person can no longer participate in making his or her own health decisions.

Funeral and Burial Arrangements

Many funeral arrangements can be made in advance, and some individuals who know they are dying may want to take an active role in the planning. Even if you will be doing this on your own, a lot of information can be gathered in advance. This is not an uncommon practice, and the people within the funeral industry will be happy to guide you—that is their job.

Buying a Plot. There are good reasons for buying a burial plot ahead of time. The family is spared having to deal with this in a rush, careful consideration can be given to location, and it can be cost-effective. Other family members can be included, but make sure everyone is informed of the arrangement. My father bought an extra plot for me, but I never knew until I happened to ask.

Vicki laughs when she tells how her husband, who has lived in a precarious state of health for years, tackled the issue of burial plots:

> He went out one day to find burial places for us, and he bought *twelve* because they were cheaper that way! I said to him, "We have no children. My family is well provided for. Your family is well provided for. What are we going to do with them?" He ordered this magnificent granite monument, had it engraved "Smythe and Friends," and began giving places away to people who did not have a place to be buried. At least he is looking at the future with that sense of humor.

Funeral Home. Simon chose a funeral home a month before Claire's death. He checked into costs for burial versus cremation and made decisions about autopsy, embalming, viewing, casket, cosmetics, and clothing. "I had the whole thing mapped out," he says. "It's just logical to plan these things if you know somebody is going to die." Making some decisions in advance saves you having to make them quickly when you are in shock and under severe emotional strain. You have time to explore all of your options instead of being pressured into expensive arrangements when you haven't the strength to resist. A good funeral director guides you through the entire process with gentleness and sensitivity. There is nothing morbid about any of it, but there are dozens of details to be worked out. You need the experience of a professional to help you to get through the logistics.

You can even plan the service. I know a man who has had his own funeral planned for years; he has bought the plot, chosen the music and the Scripture readings, and left instructions about dress and viewing. It has become something of a family joke, but that family will one day be grateful that all of those decisions have been made for them.

Disbursement of Possessions. A family can be torn apart over the distribution of family heirlooms—or even inexpensive items with great sentimental value—if no forethought is given to this matter. I know several people who have not spoken to a brother or sister for twenty or thirty years because of bad feelings generated during the settling of the estate.

The options available for disbursement of possessions are limited only by your creativity. Some people make detailed wills. Others take great pleasure in personally giving their special belongings to friends and family rather than having them distributed after their death. A few set up very elaborate lotteries or other procedures for their children to follow.

You and your spouse can sit down together and make up a list that at least covers many smaller items. Ask family members now what is important to them. Don't forget about friends who might like something as a remembrance. One of my close friends coveted a particular purse of mine and used to jokingly say, "Beverly, when you die, I don't want you to leave me any money. All I want is your purse." Had I not finally given it to her for her birthday, I most certainly would have listed it in my will!

Organ Donations. Many people find it immensely helpful to know that their death or the death of a loved one can extend life for someone else. Because Michael was wait-listed for a kidney transplant but never could have waited as long as it would have taken to get one when so many younger people were ahead of him, I learned that we need to raise the consciousness of the public on this matter. In order to be listed as a donor myself, I recently got a new driver's license—the first place authorities will look if I should die suddenly. If organ donations are of interest to you and your spouse (the feasibility of such a move may depend on the illness), get the necessary forms signed in advance and keep them in an easily accessible location. The will is not an appropriate place because the reading of it occurs too long after death to make donations possible.

Obituary. Begin accumulating biographical data so that the obituary can be quickly put together when the time comes. Some people go so far as to prepare one ahead of time, and even the dying person may want to take part. What I did when Michael died was call his office and have them dig out a copy of his bio. You can also decide in advance about flowers or donations to a favorite organization so that your preference can be included in the obituary. Michael's friends and colleagues donated so many thousands of dollars to the Georgia Diabetes Association that a "Michael Kievman Fund" was established in his honor.

Certification of Death. Check out state and local laws regarding the certification of death so you immediately know whom to call. You might need to call your doctor, the sheriff, the county coroner or medical examiner, or the police. If you haven't investigated this in advance, a call to a funeral home will tell you all you need to know.

People to Call. Make a list of names and telephone numbers in the order in which people should be contacted, and consider delegating someone to help with this difficult and time-consuming task when the time comes. Don't forget to notify your husband or wife's college or industry publications and your hometown newspaper.

When Death Arrives

Shelly was only thirty-four when she died from diabetes. Jack wasn't at all prepared, even though Shelly had been on a downhill slide for some time:

> I never did realize it was going to be that way, and Shelly didn't either. Even up to the last week, it never crossed her mind that she was going to die young. She honestly thought she'd live to be eighty-seven years old, like her grandmother. I never thought she'd live to be old like that, but I was really shocked. I thought she had maybe five more years, three years, something like that. It really happened suddenly.

Simon, on the other hand, was well prepared when Claire finally succumbed to cirrhosis:

> I went to wake her up, and when I touched her hand she was cold and stiff. I said, "Whoa, boy, it's over. It's happened." It was a shock . . . and yet you're expecting it . . . and in a way it's a relief.
>
> I started the whole process working, like you push a button for the dishwasher. That may sound cold and callous, but that's exactly what you have to do. No panic or running around or screaming or boohooing or whatever. I had a list of everybody I wanted to call, and within an hour it was all done.

I was in Nashville when Michael died. He'd been getting progressively weaker for the previous month, but I had no way of knowing that this wasn't just part of his up-and-down cycle of chronic illness, so I felt safe in going on a short business trip. When the secretary interrupted my meeting to say, "Your son Mark is on the phone; he needs to speak with you *now*," I knew what had happened.

It was time. We all knew what was next, and it wasn't pretty. Next came more amputations, more hospitalizations, and probably blindness. I think everyone felt happy for Michael, knowing what he would have had to face. As my son Steve said, "The last few weeks Michael was like a did not transfer utilities into my name until after Michael's death. I then created a note that said: "It is with sadness that I inform you that my husband passed away on [date]. Would you please change your records into my name." I included a copy with every bill I paid.

My clients were wonderful. They circled around me in a private office, and together we prayed. The president of the company and two senior vice-presidents took me to the airport, made my reservation, and did not leave me for the hour I had to wait. I was in a state of semi-shock, but when I got on the plane I immediately began to take control of this new situation. This was not the time to cry. To me it was important to find a private place before I could lose control, and in the meantime there were countless things that had to be done.

I took out my notepad and my address book and began making a list of the people who needed to be called, and I decided who was going to do the calling. Michael would have laughed had he seen me. He would have accused me of delegating, which I was so good at—anything to get out of doing the actual work. But that's what my business personality was all about, and that habit didn't stop when I crossed over into my personal life.

Was I prepared? Yes, in an intellectual sense. Did I think he was going to die? No, or I wouldn't have been away. And I don't think you're ever prepared in the emotional sense. It's always a shock.

Because of my innate need to organize, I was able to begin sifting through the details that lay ahead of me like building blocks strewn helter-skelter across the landscape, putting together the new structure that was to be my life. But, just as when I was preparing to bring Michael home from the hospital after he'd lost his second leg, I kept wishing for a blueprint to help me find my way. Long after it would have done me any good, I found the blueprint I had longed for, a checklist compiled by the accounting firm of Deloitte Haskins & Sells. With their permission I would like to pass it along to you.

Checklist to Use in the Event of Death

1. Telephone a friend to spend the next few hours with you if you are alone. Shock and trauma can take unexpected forms.
2. Make an appointment with a funeral director to discuss funeral arrangements. Ask for several copies of your spouse's death certificate, which you will need for your spouse's employer, life insurance companies, and legal procedures.
3. Locate the family's important papers. Get as many as you can together and continue the gathering process over the next weeks.
4. You should be aware that certain *jointly held* assets, such as safe deposit boxes and checking or savings accounts, may be frozen as soon as the bank or other institution involved becomes aware that one of the joint owners has died. Thus, although such assets are intended to pass to the surviving spouse outside the normal probate process, actual possession of such assets may be delayed pending a court order releasing them. Such an order may depend on satisfying inheritance or estate tax officials that the estate owns other assets adequate to pay any potential estate or inheritance tax.
5. Make an appointment with your tax advisor and attorney to review your spouse's will and to discuss any state and federal death taxes payable.
6. Notify your Inheritance Tax Office and ask for the required forms. In many states, you must have a release from this office before company benefits or insurance benefits can be paid. (The office will be listed under your state listing in the phone book if you live in an urban area. If you do not, your tax advisor can supply you with the proper address.)
7. Telephone your spouse's employee benefits office. Tell them: your spouse's name, spouse's Social Security number, date of death, whether

death due to accident or illness; your name and address. The company can then begin to process any benefits payable immediately.

8. If your spouse was eligible for Medicare, notify them, giving them the same information as in #7 above.
9. Notify Social Security of the death. Claims may be expedited if you go to the nearest Social Security office in person to sign a claim for survivor's benefit. Look for the address under U.S. Government in the telephone book.
10. If you need emergency cash before insurance claims are paid, a cash advance may be made from any life insurance benefits to which you are entitled.
11. If your spouse was in the service, notify the Veterans Administration. You may be eligible for death or disability benefits.
12. In a small ledger keep track of all money you spend. These figures will be needed for tax returns.
13. Remember that you are in a highly emotional state. Avoid contracting for anything, and avoid spending or lending large sums of money.
14. Contact your accountant or financial advisors for an appointment to discuss updated planning.

After a Few Weeks:

The paperwork will begin to diminish. You can then take the opportunity to make any necessary changes in ownership registration for:

- Auto registration
- Stock, bonds, investments
- Residence
- Boat
- Savings and checking accounts. (You may wish to open a joint account with another member of your family.)

- Charge accounts
- Safe deposit box

You may wish to make a new will.

While there is much to do, *any major decisions should be deferred for at least a year.* You will be working your way through the grieving process without the proper perspective to ensure sound judgment. If you can possibly avoid it, *don't* sell the house, *don't* move in with the children, *don't* change jobs. There will be plenty of time in the future for establishing your new life.

Location of Papers and Records

	Safe Deposit Box	Office	Residence
Wills			
Trust agreements			
Powers of attorney			
Burial instructions			
Cemetery deed			
Safe combination			
Employment benefits			
Employment contracts			
Stock plans			
Stock options			
Pension records			
Social Security records			
Life insurance			
Property insurance			
Casualty insurance			
Birth certificate			
Passport			
Naturalization papers			
Military discharge			
Marriage certificate			
Family personal papers			

	Safe Deposit Box	Office	Residence
Partnership agreements			
Checking account records			
Savings account passbook			
Credit card records			
Certificates of deposit			
Record of investment portfolio			
Stock certificates			
Bonds			
Mutual fund shares			
Tax returns			
Real estate titles and deeds			
Title insurance			
Mortgage papers			
Notes payable			
Notes receivable			
Ownership records:			
Auto			
Boat			
Recreational property			
Maintenance papers:			
Home			
Auto			
Other			
Addresses of relatives and friends			
Lists of organization memberships			

Important Names and Numbers

Social Security Number _____
EMPLOYER _____
Address _____
_____

Phone _____
ACCOUNTANT _____
Address _____

Phone _____
ATTORNEY _____
Address _____

Phone _____
STOCKBROKER _____
Address _____

Phone _____
INSURANCE AGENT _____
Address _____

Phone _____
GUARDIAN _____
Address _____

Phone _____
CHILDREN'S GUARDIAN _____
Address _____

Phone _____
TRUST OFFICER _____
Address _____

Phone _____
FINANCIAL COUNSELOR _____
Address _____

Completing the Circle

A lot of this book has been about communication. A marriage, after all, is an agreement to live together for the rest of your lives, and you can't do that comfortably without working together, without reassessing the constantly shifting marital balance.

Nothing is sadder than two people, who have chosen each other as lifelong companions, facing an occasion as momentous as death without talking about it. Because they can't verbalize their fears and share their concerns, they withdraw, little by little, into their own separate worlds. Simon and Claire chose this route:

> We never talked about it. We kind of played a game, even though we knew it was just a matter of months. We'd talk about how the liver could repair itself, that kind of nonsense, what we'd do when the boys got home, getting the bathroom done. She went and bought a bunch of wallpaper and took the medicine cabinet out of the bathroom and was going to redo it all. Those rolls of wallpaper are still sitting there.

Simon and Claire made a game out of skirting the issue of death, and yet when Simon once hit too close to home by saying, "It's going to be interesting to see what kind of grandchildren the boys give us," the game lost its fun, and he was cut off with a curt remark. When Claire died, she was alone.

When Michael died he was also alone (in our bed, that is) but there was a difference because he knew that I was with him in spirit. Every conversation we had at that time was complete, which was terribly important to both of us. The night before he died, as I did every night when I was away, I called. We had a wonderful conversation. I told him I loved him, and he told me he loved me.

I did not experience any If Onlys: if only I'd called last night . . . if only I hadn't fussed at him for not drinking his juice . . . if only I hadn't gone on that trip to Nashville . . . When Michael died, he was at peace in his soul and in his heart—and so was I.

The days after the death were far harder on the children than they were on me, for two reasons. First, I was consumed by the details of arranging the funeral and sorting out the business end of our affairs. Second, I had already done much of my grieving before Michael died. *With chronic illness, there are little good-byes all along the way as each half of the team says good-bye to the part of the marriage that is no more.* That final good-bye is just one more.

A week after the funeral I felt a need to make a final farewell toast to Michael and to the life we had shared. For a setting I chose our dock on Lake Lanier, a spot that had come to represent tranquility in the midst of fear and sadness, hope during bouts of despair, and beauty that distracted us from his disfigurement. It might now become a melancholy place, but I was certain that the ducks Michael had befriended there would never let that happen. At sunset I took my trusty box of Kleenex, a glass of wine, and food for the ducks and strolled down to the dock. As I stared at the beauty of the November evening and basked in the tranquility that was symbolic of the peace Michael had at last found, I saw Betsy, Knothead Jr., No Name, Lucybird, and a gaggle of their friends heading my way. Michael would have been pleased.

BEAR IN MIND:

Don't be afraid to talk about the end that is coming. Many individuals find that death is easier to face if they are allowed to take part in planning the ceremony of passing.

Prepare for terminal illness. By taking certain legal steps in advance, you can eliminate many of the complications that arise when a member of a family dies.

Be sure there is a valid will or living trust. It is astonishing how many people are unaware of the importance of having a will.

Consult a lawyer. It is well worth whatever fees you pay now for legal and financial advice for the money and trouble that can be saved in the long run.

Talk openly with your spouse. Nothing is sadder than two people, who have chosen each other as lifelong companions, facing an occasion as momentous as death without talking about it.

Letting go is a gradual process. With chronic illness, there are little good-byes all along the way as each half of the team says good-bye to the part of the marriage that is no more.

Epilogue

M ichael's life was in the film and broadcasting business; he was an expert in television programming. A TV or motion picture script is written with a story line that focuses on an event or a moment in time. Most, however, focus on someone's life. The story line is the plot and usually has one or two stars.

Our children—indeed, most people forty years old or younger—have grown up in an era when television dominated their lives. Subtly, they have been conditioned to believe that life stories come in thirty- or sixty-minute time blocks, and even sad stories must have implied happy endings. The life stories in this book show that is not necessarily true.

Michael wrote his own script, and I have the privilege and awesome responsibility to edit it, to select the moment in time the story begins . . . and ends.

The story begins at a piano bar in Atlanta, Georgia, in the mid-1970s. The story ends in a broken-down, old boat in Grand Cayman at sunset as our six children, Michael's sister, and I respect his wish that his ashes be scattered into the Caribbean Sea he loved so much.

The closing moment in the script shows that old boat leaving the dock, filled to capacity with eight people riding in absolute silence. It was a perfect evening to go out for a sunset boat ride as we had done countless times in the past. The sky was crystal clear, the wind was gentle, and the turquoise water lapped playfully against the boat. Each of us had reddened eyes, and some of us were crying silently, the tears rolling down our cheeks. Michele clutched the urn. None of us had ever been through this experience before.

From time to time someone would be moved to speak, while the rest of us listened in silence, replaying in our own minds precious moments of our life together with Michael. What episodes did each of us review over and over? Was it the picture of sadness with Michael in the hospital a year before, hooked up to tubes everywhere, lying gaunt and listless after his second amputation? Was it of Mike the executive in his office, tossing pencils at the ceiling? Or gentle Grandpa Mike sound asleep in a chair holding his two-year-old grandson, also sound asleep? Certainly it was the Michael of a few weeks ago, proudly and independently riding his "tricycle" and feeding his pet ducks and geese.

A script of chronic illness doesn't have a happy ending; the closest thing in the real-life script is that the pain and sadness are over. We hope, pray, and believe that our loved one has found peace.

As we sat in that old boat in Cayman Sound watching the sunset, I thought of the closing moments of Michael's script. There is a song in *The King and I* that expresses beautifully a truth we all need to remember. When you love someone, that person need not be perfect. But that person has dreams that are important, and you defend those dreams to other people. In times of illness it is vital to let your loved one know that his or her spirit is still strong and that you love and believe in that person. I will always be thankful that we were able to let Michael know of our love and belief.

Flash back to April 7, 1987, the night of Michael's phenomenal surprise party. Camera pans the room to show 250 people in the grand ballroom of the hotel paying tribute to a tough son-of-a-gun who survived his near-death only four months earlier. Fast forward the evening of joy and roasting to the moment the camera closes in on the star for a few words. No one present will *ever* forget the moment he said:

"And I don't know if I will ever stand up again—much less walk—for the rest of my life, but I want you to know that I'm going to try and I am going to do it . . . right . . . *now.*"

Camera pulls back to show Michael put the microphone down and, as though nothing wrong in the world had ever happened, rise out of his wheelchair, stand up, and raise his arms in the most victorious moment of his life.

A story of courage.

A story of love.

Fade to black.

Suggested Readings

Self-Healing

Cousins, Norman. *Anatomy of an Illness as Perceived by the Patient: Reflections on Healing and Regeneration* (New York: W. W. Norton & Co., 1979). In this remarkable book Norman Cousins explores the avenues to self-healing through the power of the mind. Struck down by an imminently terminal disease, he discontinued all drugs and left the hospital to devote all of his energy to making himself well. A good introduction to the principles of holistic medicine.

Siegel, Bernie S. *Love, Medicine and Miracles* (New York: Harper & Row, 1986). By breaking down the doctor-patient barrier and opening his heart to his patients, this surgeon discovered that love heals. In his work with exceptional patients who have learned how to heal themselves, Dr. Siegel teaches us lessons that every patient and doctor should know.

Home Nursing

Coombs, Jan. *Living with the Disabled: You Can Help* (New York: Sterling Publishing Co., 1984). A positive, forward-looking book aimed at achieving full personal potential. Information on insurance, plus federal, state, and community programs. Provides an extensive list of organizations for specific disabilities and services.

Covell, Mara Brand. *The Home Alternative to Hospitals and Nursing Homes* (New York: Rawson Associates, 1983). Written by a medical journalist who has also had personal experience in caring for a family member. Provides many practical ideas for improvising and for converting existing household supplies rather than buying or renting expensive equipment. In-depth sections on resources, diet, and nursing skills.

Friedman, Jo-Ann. *Home Health Care: A Complete Guide for Patients and Their Families* (New York and London: W. W. Norton & Co., 1986). Guidelines for preparing the home and for dealing with Medicare, Medicaid, and insurance companies. Many charts, worksheets, and questionnaires for assessment of the feasibility of home care and of finding the best home-care specialists. List of tips for daily living. Separate chapters on common health problems. Extensive resource list organized according to type of disease or disability.

Hastings, Diana. *The Complete Guide to Home Nursing*, ed. Helen Maule (Woodbury, NY: Barron's, 1986). A virtual encyclopedia of nursing care. Describes nursing skills in great detail, with abundant illustrations. Covers the home care needed for many specific illnesses and conditions. Includes a section on first aid.

Horne, Jo. *Helping an Aging Loved One* (Washington, DC: American Association of Retired Persons; sold by Scott, Foresman and Co., 1985).

Mace, Nancy L., and Rabins, Peter V. *The 36-Hour Day*. While this is primarily a family guide for dealing with Alzheimer's disease, it would be of help to anyone caring for a patient with loss of normal mental functions.

Parker, Page, and Dietz, Lois N. *Nursing at Home: A Practical Guide to the Care of the Sick and the Invalid in the Home Plus Self-Help Instructions for the Patient* (New York: Crown Publishers, 1980). How-to book covering everything from moving, bathing, and exercising the patient to obtaining special equipment. Heavy emphasis upon nutrition and special diets.

Portnow, Jay, with Houtmann, Martha. *Home Care for the Elderly: A Complete Guide* (New York: McGraw-Hill, 1987).

For the Patient

Lewis, Kathleen S. *Successful Living with Chronic Illness* (Wayne, NY: Avery Publishing Group, 1985).

Pitzele, Sefra Kobrin. *We Are Not Alone: Learning to Live with Chronic Illness* (New York: Workman Publishing, 1985). From the patient's point of view, written by a woman with lupus.

Register, Cheri. *Living with Chronic Illness: Days of Patience and Passion* (New York: The Free Press, 1987). This is one of the newest and best books out on chronic illness from the patient's point of view. By sharing the emotions she faces in her battle with a defective liver, Cheri Register is an inspiration to us all.

Inspiration

Kushner, Harold S. *When Bad Things Happen to Good People* (New York: Schocken, 1981). A rabbi addresses the Why Me? issue with personal insight and compassion.

Death

Blankenship, Jayne. *In the Center of the Night: Journey Through a Bereavement* (New York: G. P. Putnam's Sons, 1984). The jacket copy says it all: "This heartrending diary of a young widow spares no details of the torturous journey through a grieving mind. No other book is as open and honest, touching upon every macabre dream and psychic experience."

Caine, Lynn. *Widow* (New York: William Morrow, 1974). To quote the book jacket: "The consequences of suppressing emotion, facing grief totally unprepared, ignorant of the dynamics of the reaction to loss, of dealing with the role of a single woman, a single parent and single provider in a coupled world, are explored here in realistic and compelling terms."

Davidson, Glen W., ed. *The Hospice: Development and Administration* (Washington, DC: Hemisphere Publishing Corp., 1975). A compilation of papers describing the history and organization of various Canadian and American hospices, problems for staff, ethics, and legal issues.

Kübler-Ross, Elisabeth. *Death: The Final Stage of Growth* (Englewood Cliffs, NJ: Prentice-Hall, 1975). Kübler-Ross puts forth the premise that only by accepting our mortality can we discover the true meaning of life. This volume includes messages for the living on better understanding and dealing with hospital staff and insurance personnel, and on working through grief and mourning. Much of this information can be of help to those dealing with chronic as well as terminal illness.

Kübler-Ross, Elisabeth. *On Death and Dying* (New York: Macmillan, 1969). The dying have much to teach doctors, nurses, clergy, and their own families. Kübler-Ross describes the five stages leading toward acceptance of one's mortality.

Kübler-Ross, Elisabeth. *Questions and Answers on Death and Dying* (New York: Macmillan, 1974).

Kübler-Ross, Elisabeth. *To Live Until We Say Good-Bye* (Englewood Cliffs, NJ: Prentice-Hall, 1978). A photographic essay on the process of death. Dr. Kübler-Ross brings four terminally ill patients and their families to an acceptance of death, while photographer Mal Warshaw captures the range of emotions involved.

Little, Deborah Whiting. *Home Care for the Dying: A Reassuring, Comprehensive Guide to Physical and Emotional Care* (Garden City, NY: Dial Press and Doubleday & Co., 1985). Geared toward the patient's comfort and relief of symptoms. Tackles emotional issues for patient, caregivers, and visitors. The chapter on physical care goes far beyond the usual explanations of nursing skills by stressing tenderness and compassion. The chapter on supplies is not the usual list, but rather a careful description of choices.

Pattison, E. Mansell. *The Experience of Dying* (Englewood Cliffs, NJ: Prentice-Hall, 1977).

Pritchard, Elizabeth R. *Home Care: Living with Dying* (New York: Columbia University Press, 1980).

Stoddard, Sandol. *The Hospice Movement: A Better Way of Caring for the Dying* (Briarcliff Manor, NY: Stein and Day, 1978). Stoddard offers a historical and philosophical look at the development of the hospice system and how and why it works.

Upson, Norma S. *When Someone You Love Is Dying* (New York: Simon & Schuster, 1986). Written expressly for the caregiver dealing with terminal illness, this thoughtful and sympathetic book discusses emotions, stress, and legal decisions. With a special chapter for nontraditional couples, it is one of few books that address the issue of AIDS. It also contains a complete bibliography of books concerning death.

Viorst, Judith. *Necessary Losses* (New York: Simon & Schuster, 1986). About loss in general, but has helpful chapters on how to deal with anger and guilt, on shifting self-images, and on mourning the loss of self as illness or disability change how things have been.

Spiritual

Holy Bible